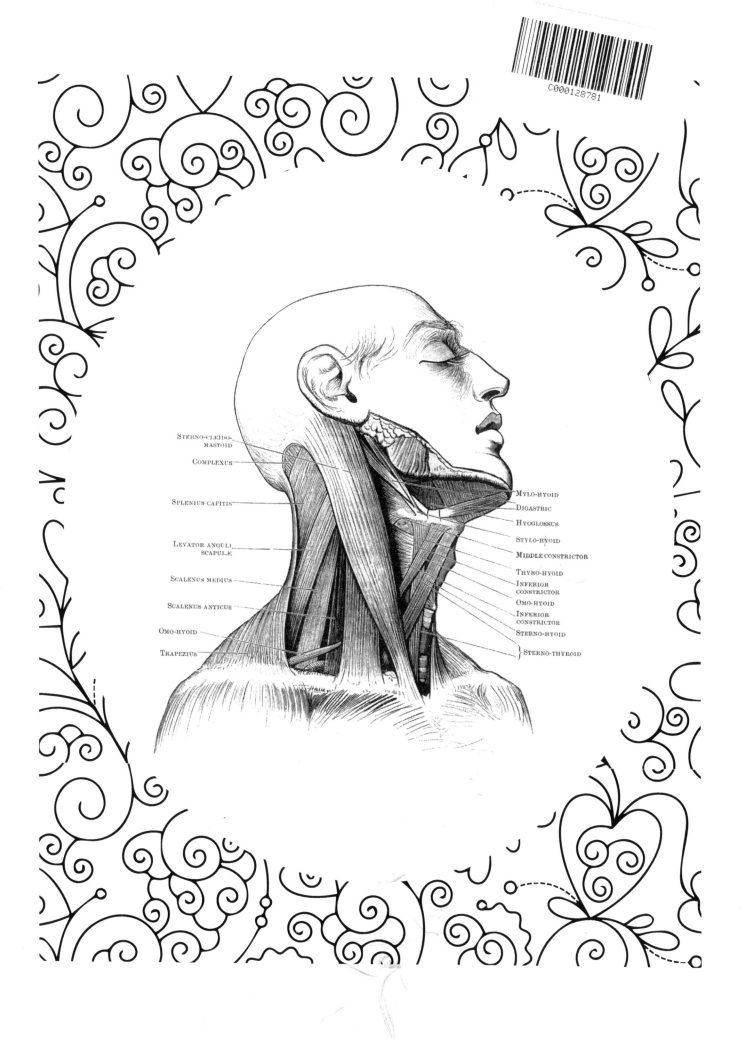

STERNO-CLEIDO-MASTOID

COMPLEXUS

SPLENIUS CAPITIS

LEVATOR ANGULI SCAPULÆ

SCALENUS MEDIUS

SCALENUS ANTICUS

OMO-HYOID

TRAPEZIUS

MYLO-HYOID

DIGASTRIC

HYOGLOSSUS

STYLO-HYOID

MIDDLE CONSTRICTOR

THYRO-HYOID

INFERIOR CONSTRICTOR

OMO-HYOID

INFERIOR CONSTRICTOR

STERNO-HYOID

STERNO-THYROID

This Book Belongs To

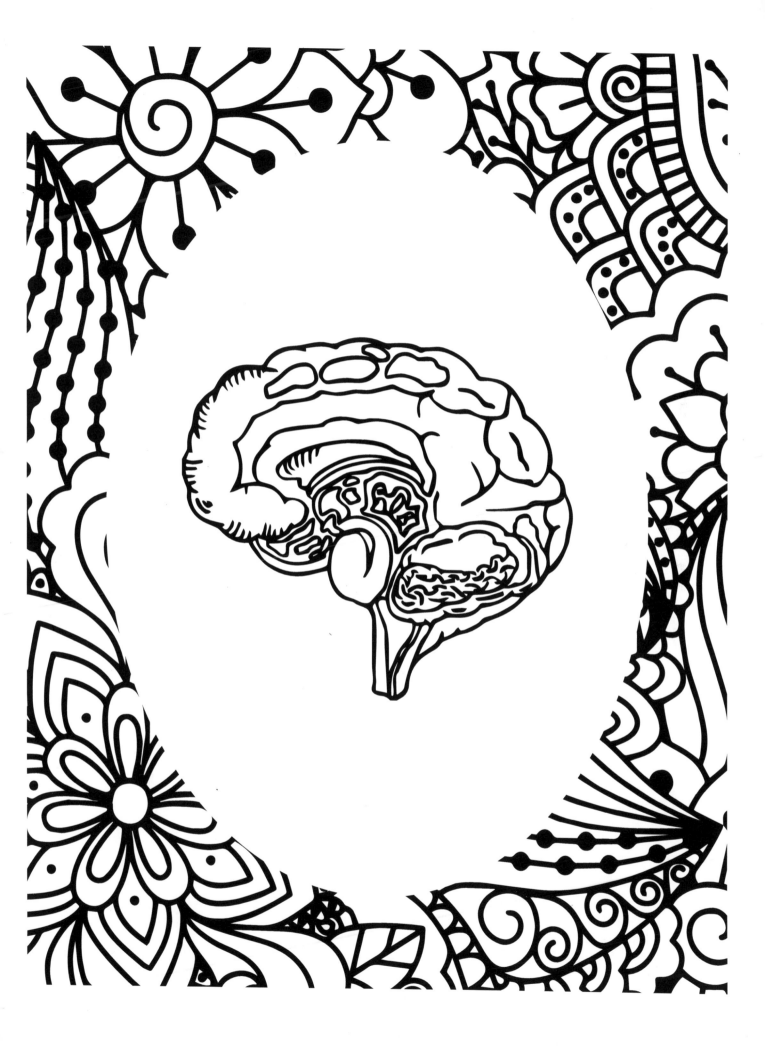

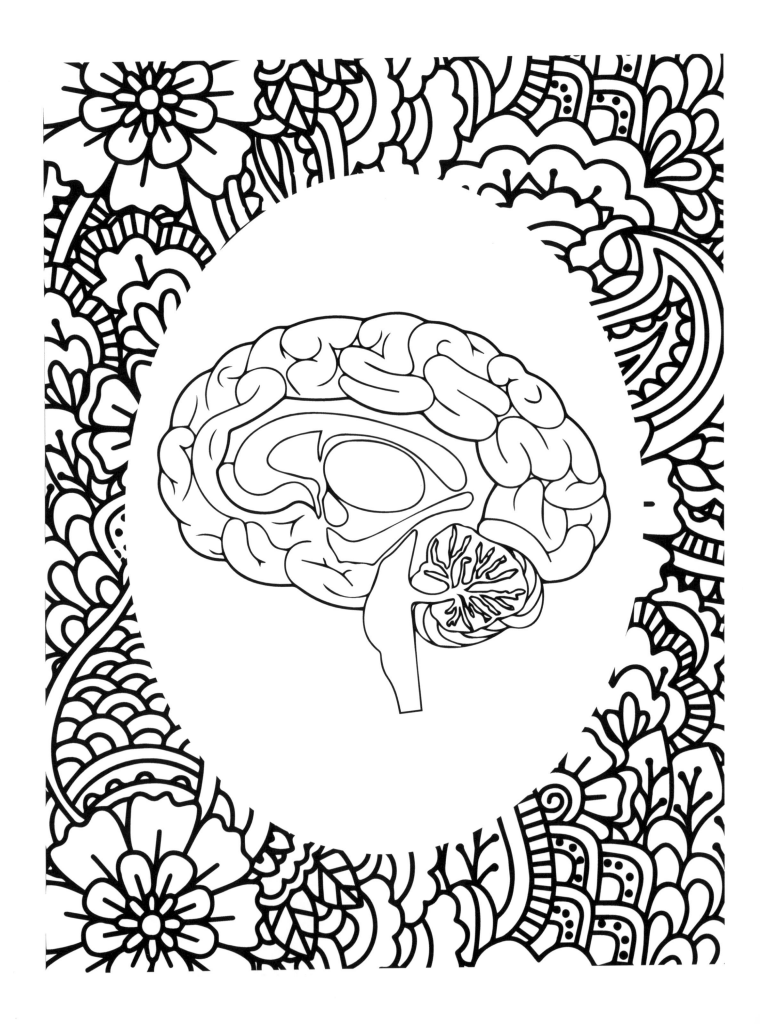

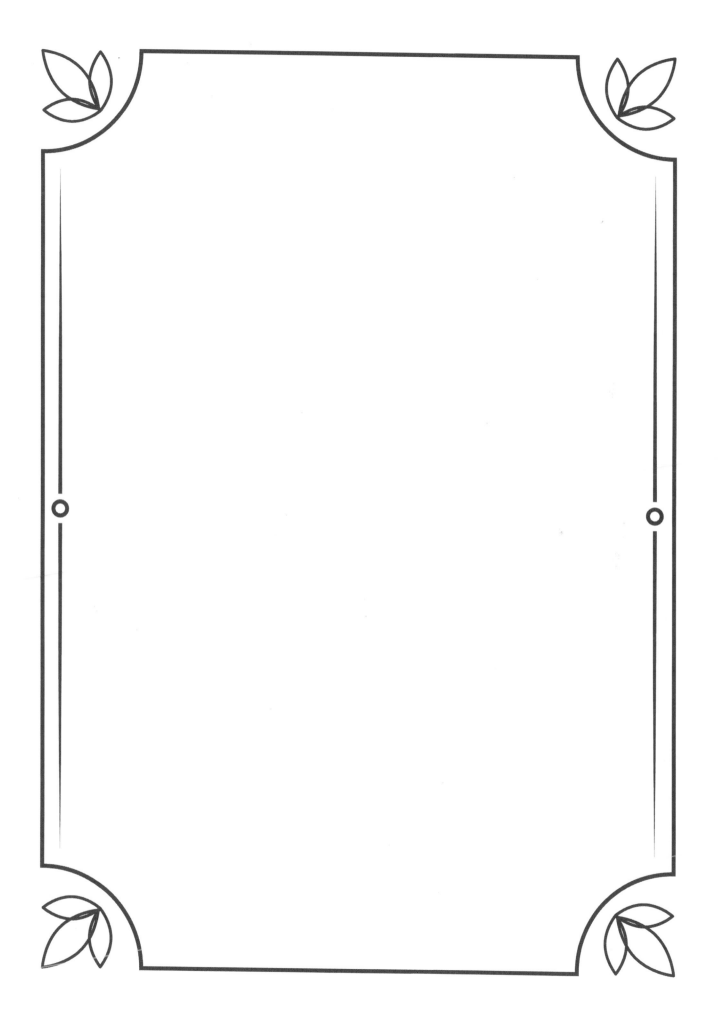

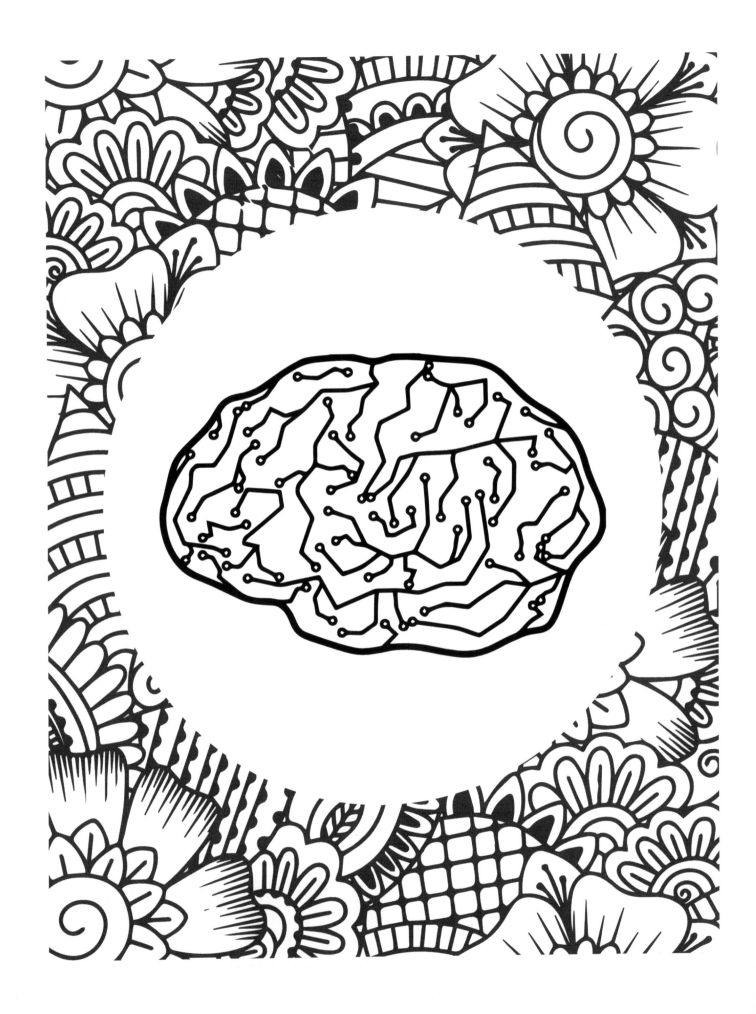

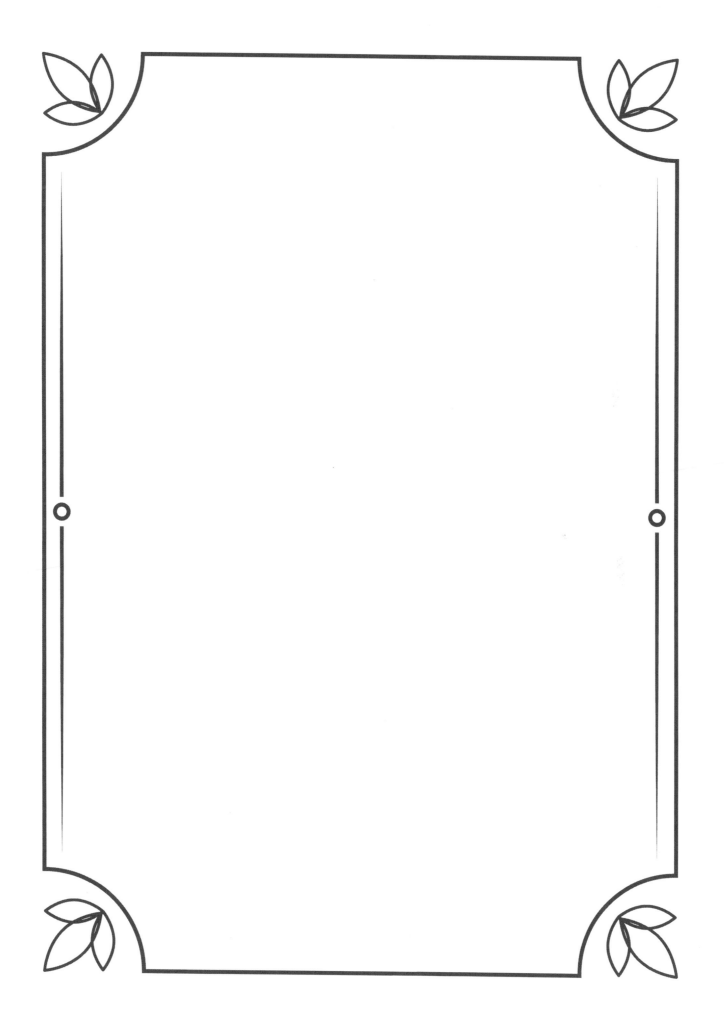

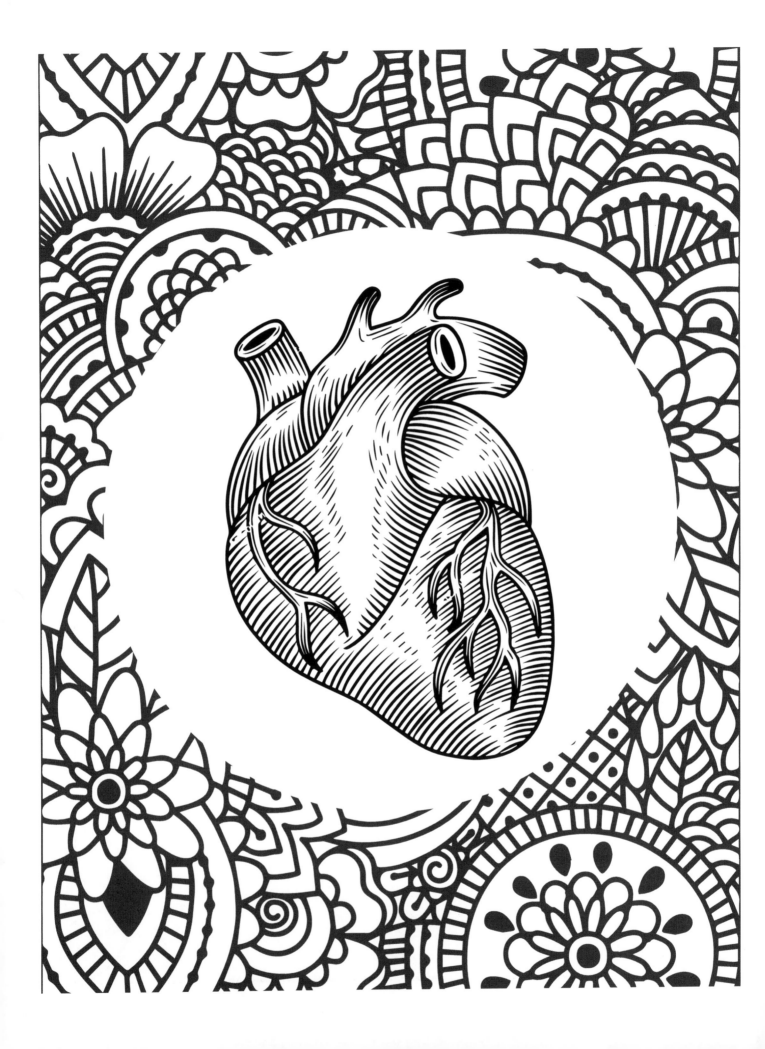

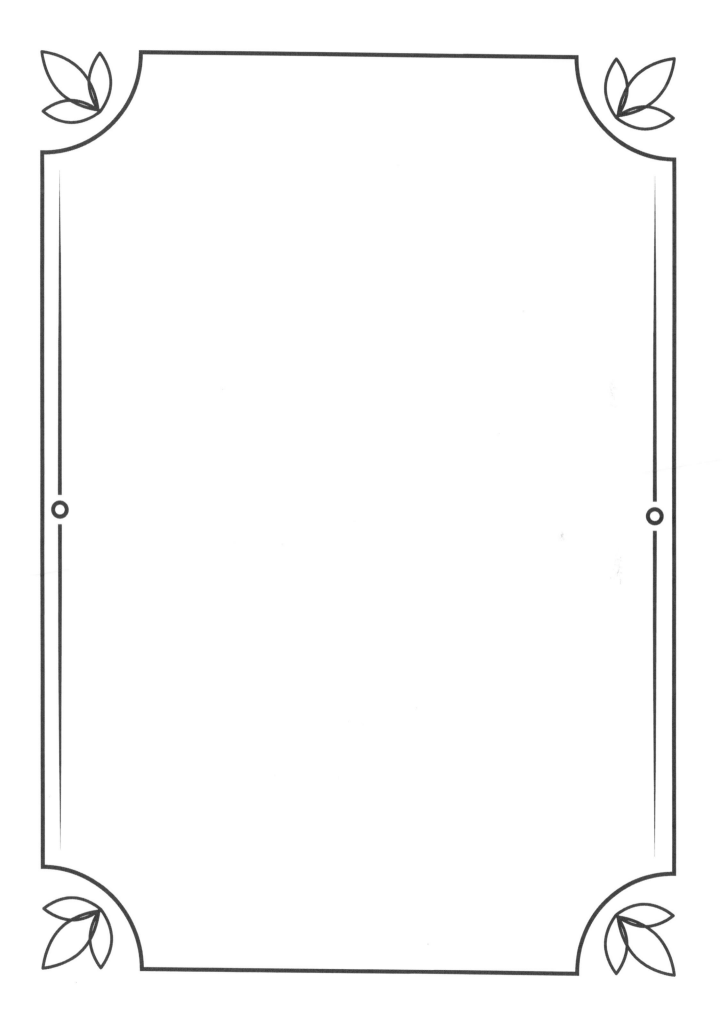

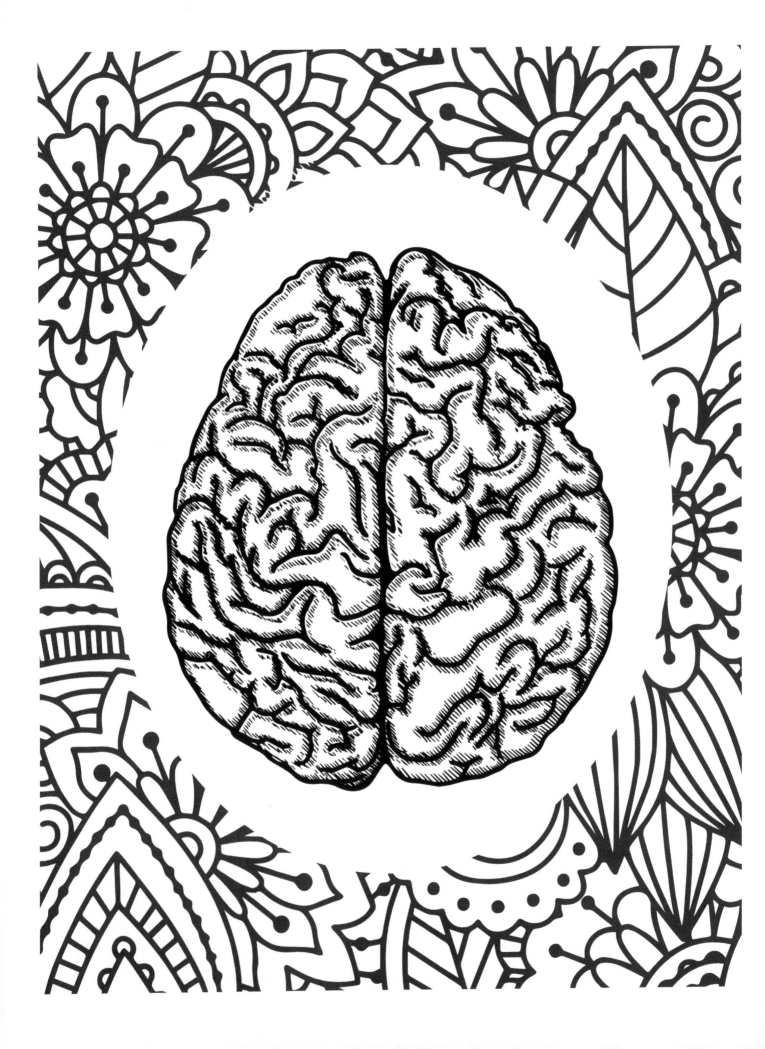

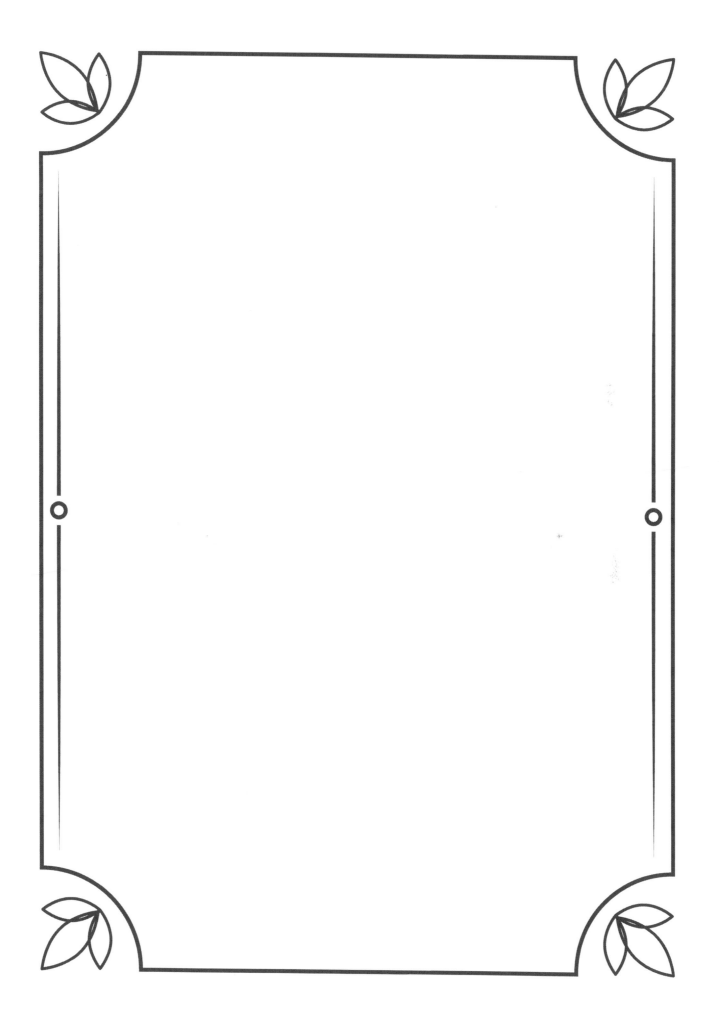

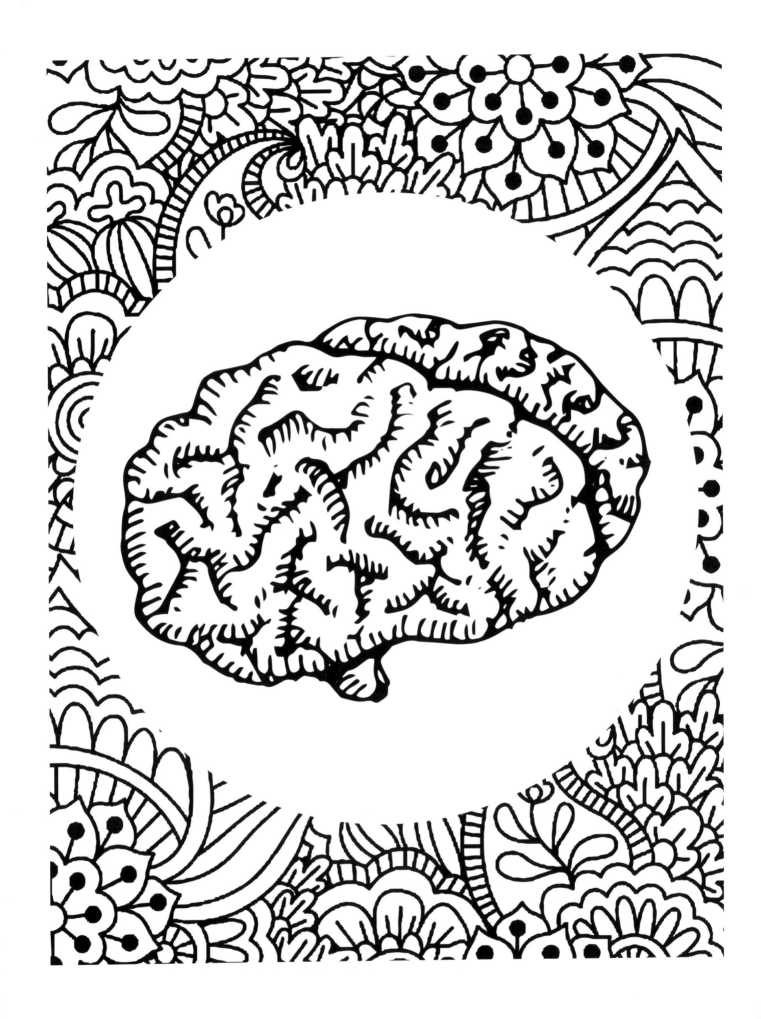

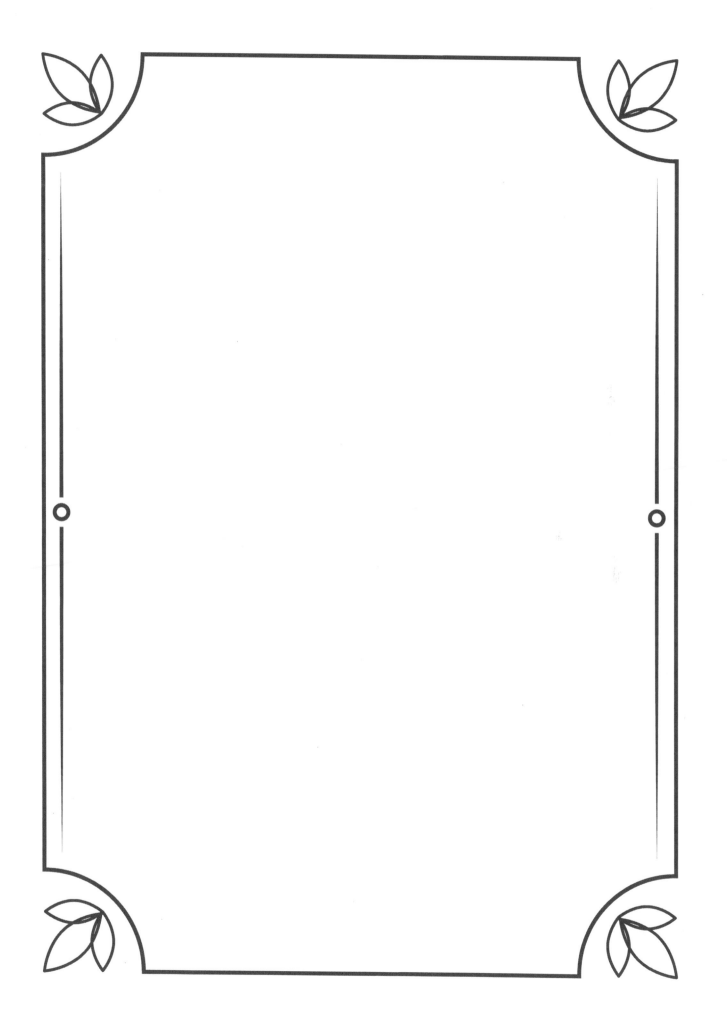

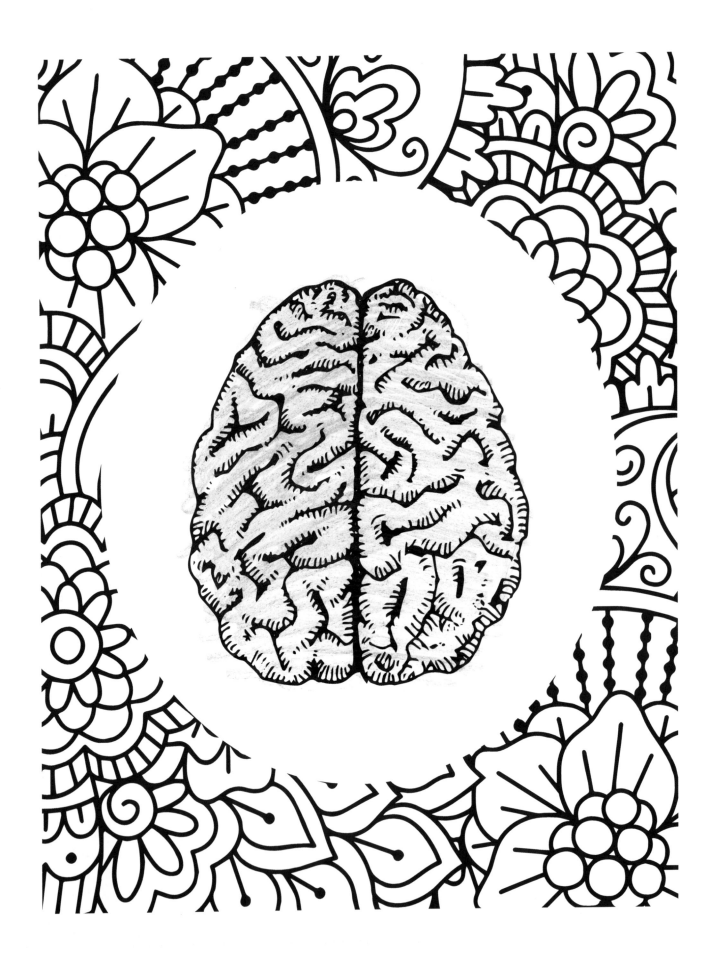

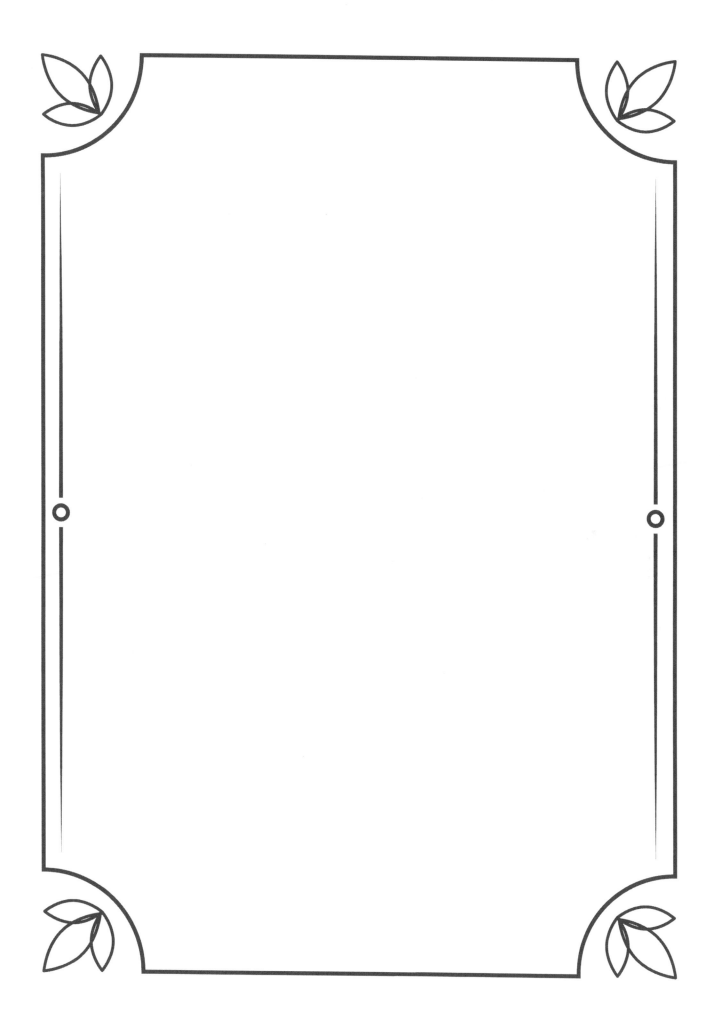

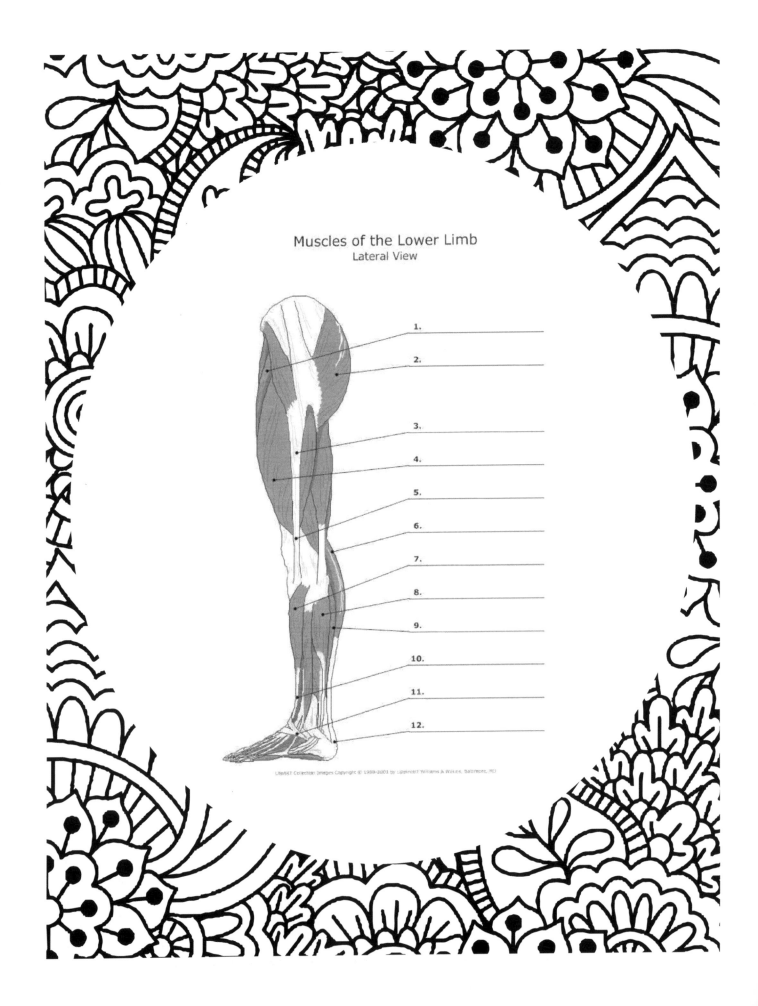

Muscles of the Lower Limb
Lateral View

1.

2.

3.

4.

5.

6.

7.

8.

9.

10.

11.

12.

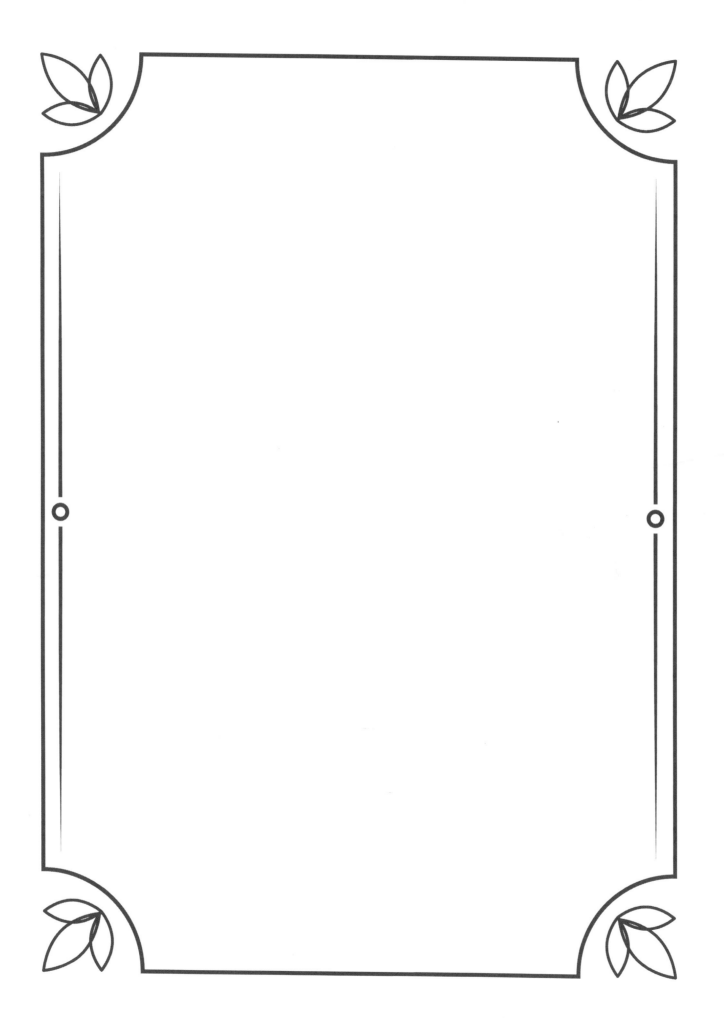

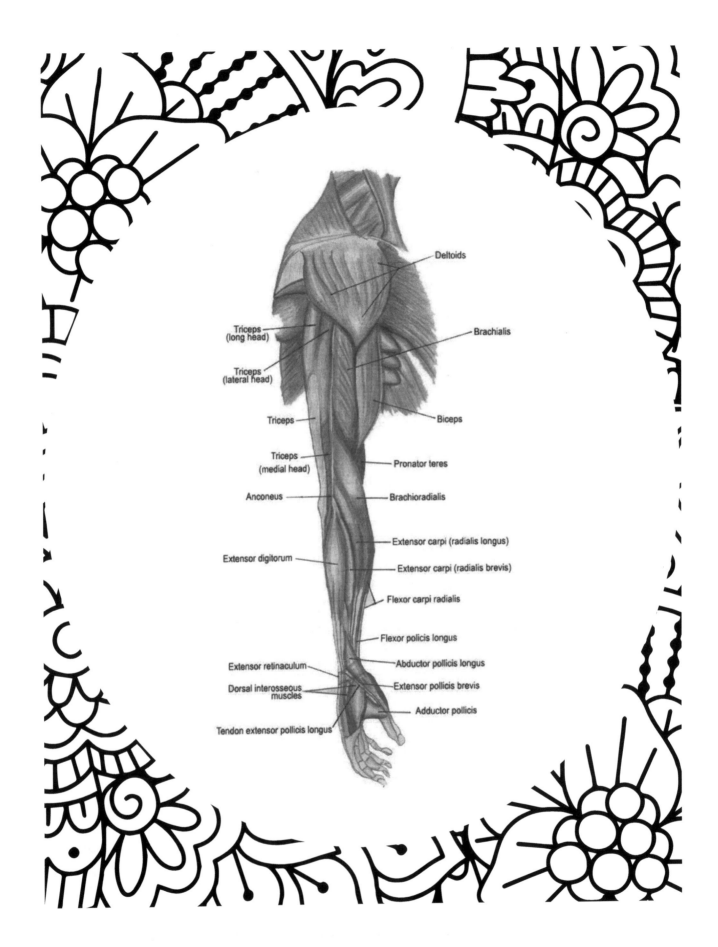

Deltoids

Triceps
(long head)

Triceps
(lateral head)

Brachialis

Triceps

Biceps

Triceps
(medial head)

Pronator teres

Anconeus

Brachioradialis

Extensor carpi (radialis longus)

Extensor digitorum

Extensor carpi (radialis brevis)

Flexor carpi radialis

Flexor policis longus

Abductor pollicis longus

Extensor retinaculum

Extensor pollicis brevis

Dorsal interosseous
muscles

Adductor pollicis

Tendon extensor pollicis longus

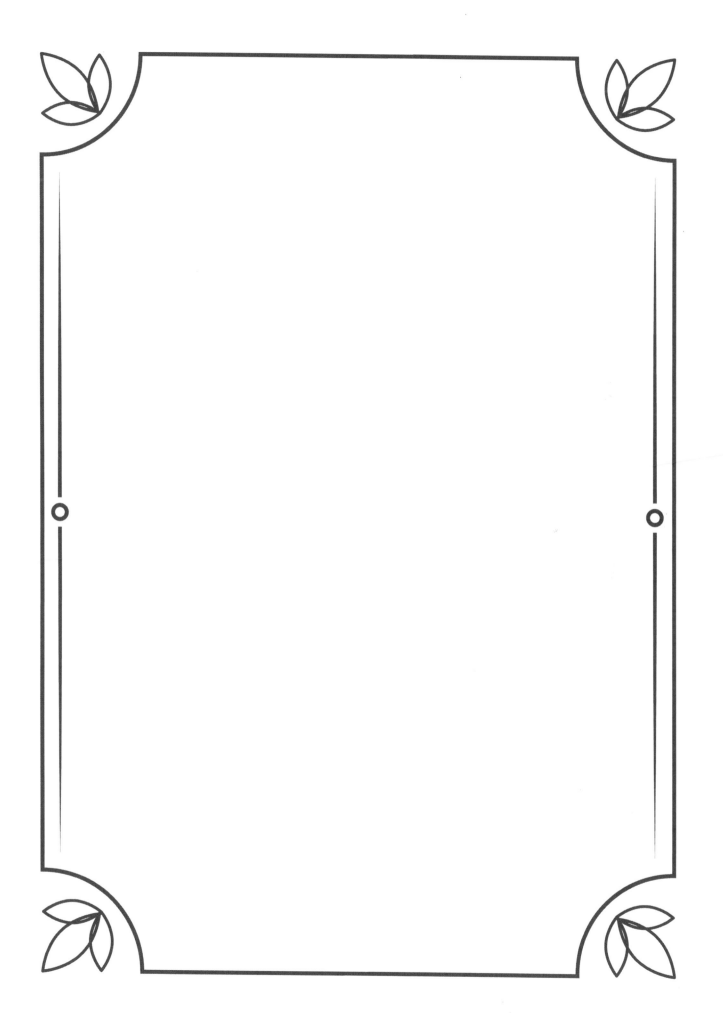

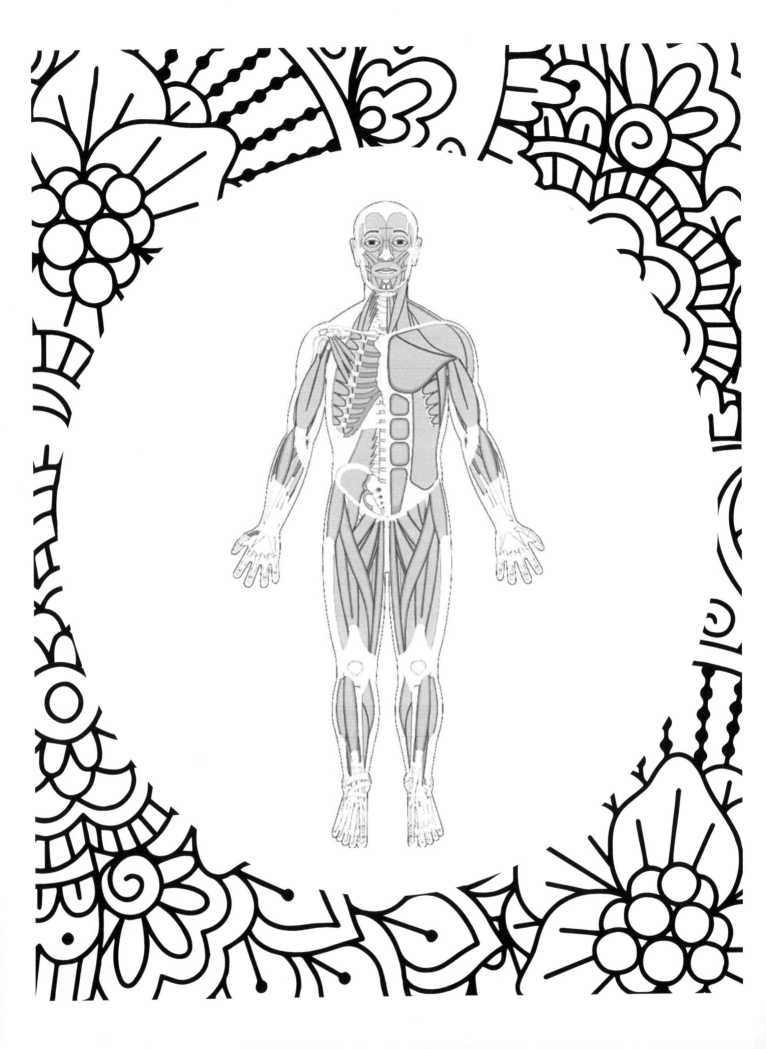

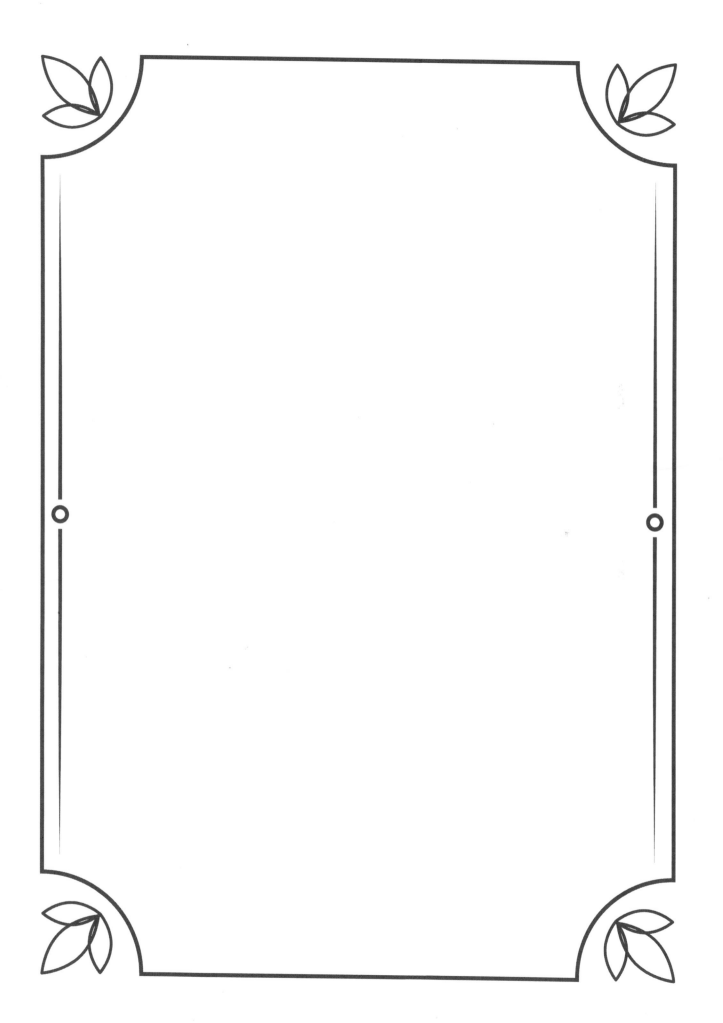

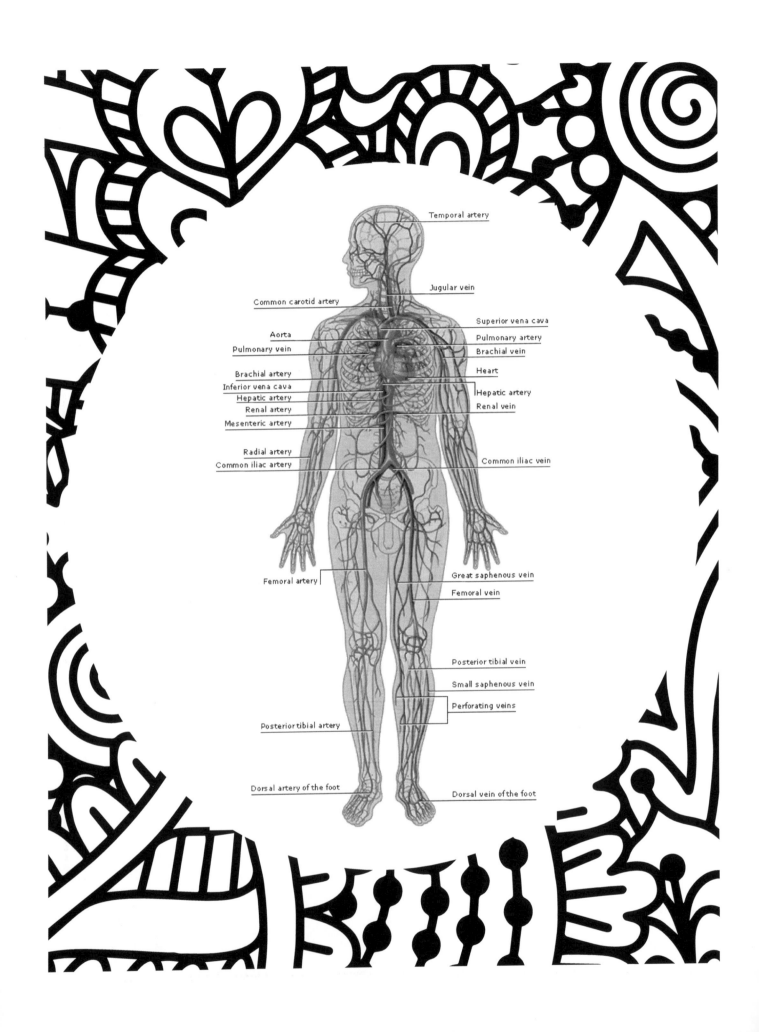

Temporal artery

Jugular vein

Common carotid artery

Superior vena cava

Aorta

Pulmonary artery

Pulmonary vein

Brachial vein

Brachial artery

Heart

Inferior vena cava

Hepatic artery

Hepatic artery

Renal vein

Renal artery

Mesenteric artery

Radial artery

Common iliac vein

Common iliac artery

Femoral artery

Great saphenous vein

Femoral vein

Posterior tibial vein

Small saphenous vein

Perforating veins

Posterior tibial artery

Dorsal artery of the foot

Dorsal vein of the foot

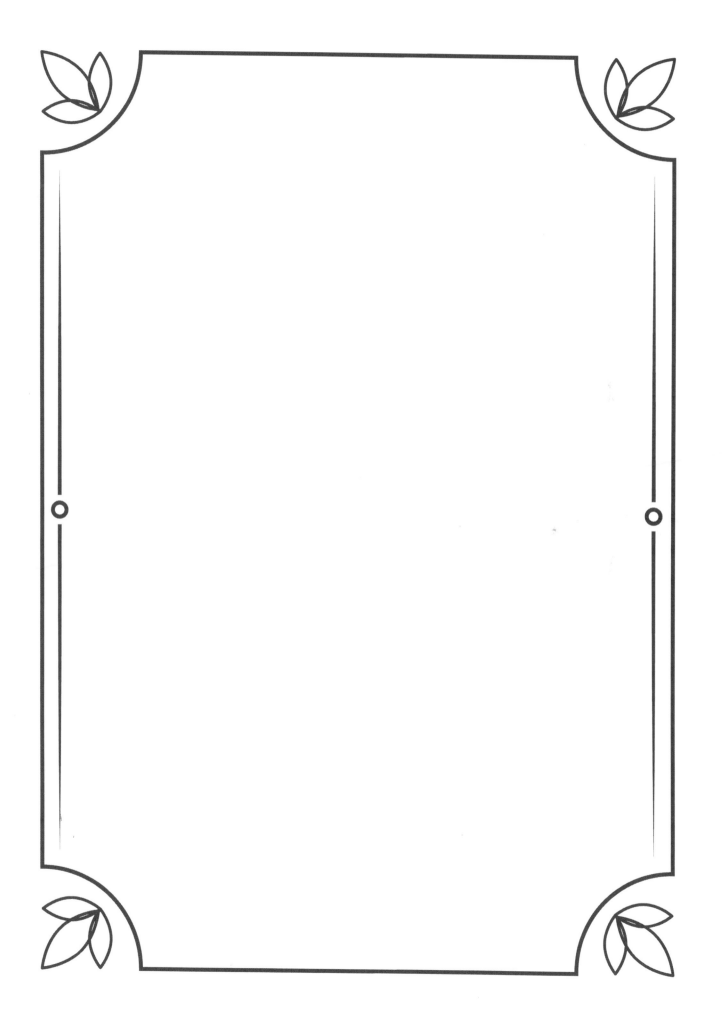

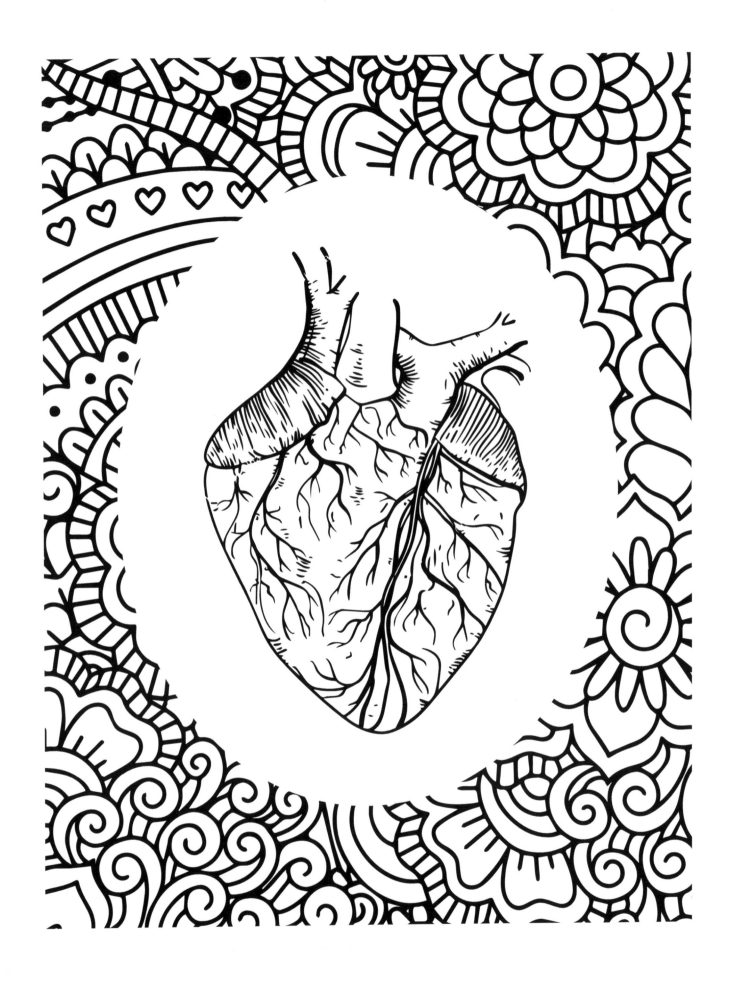

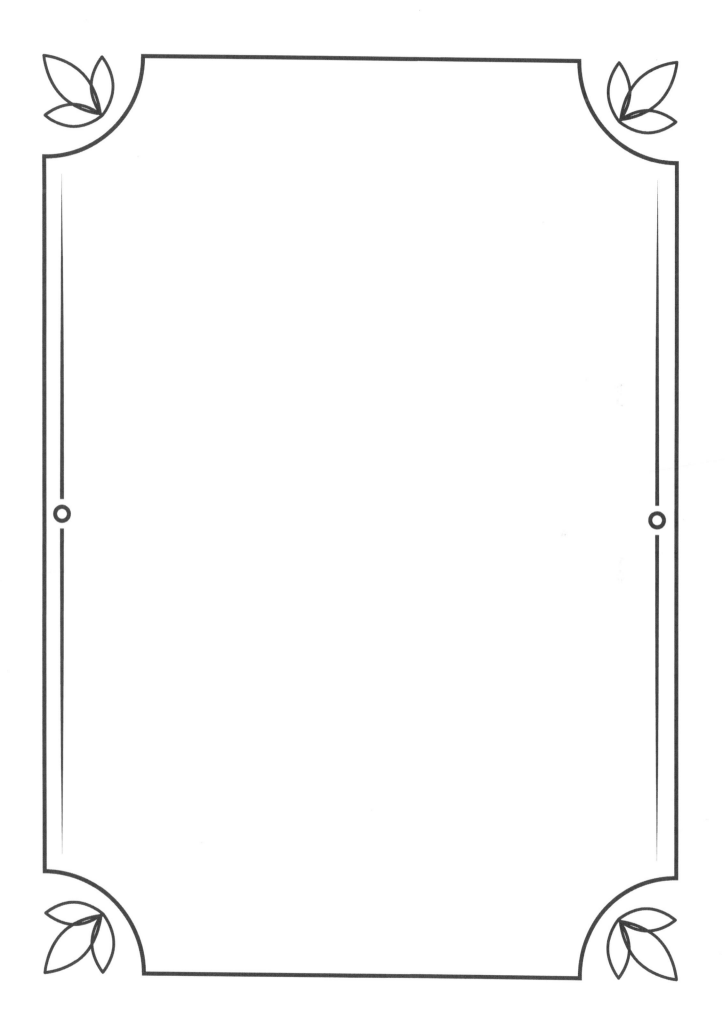

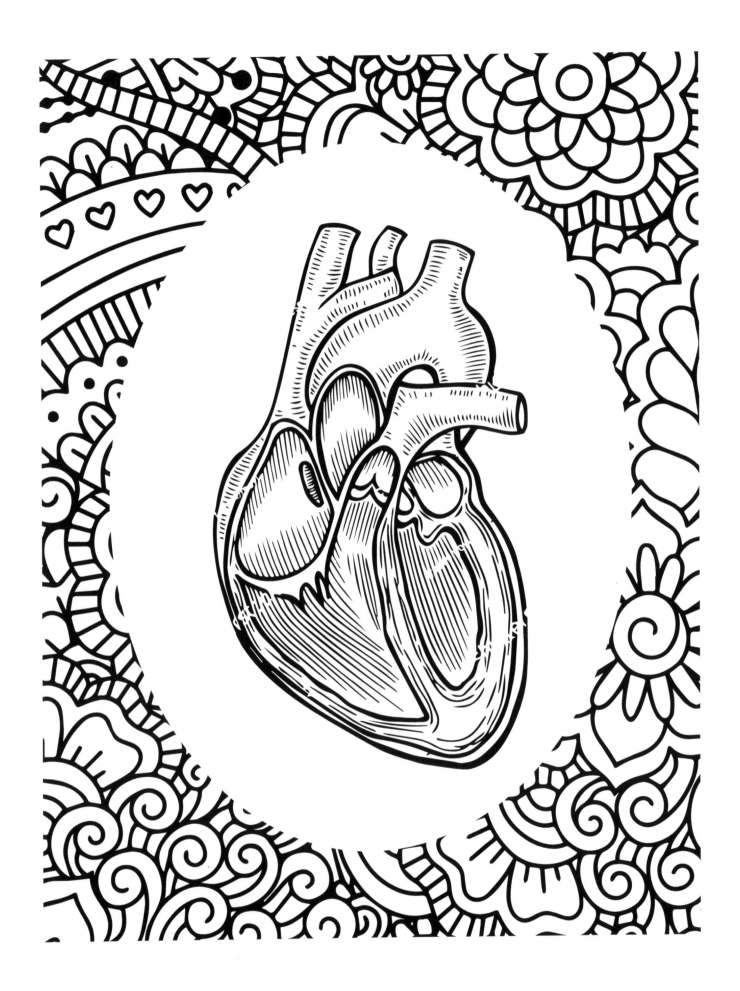

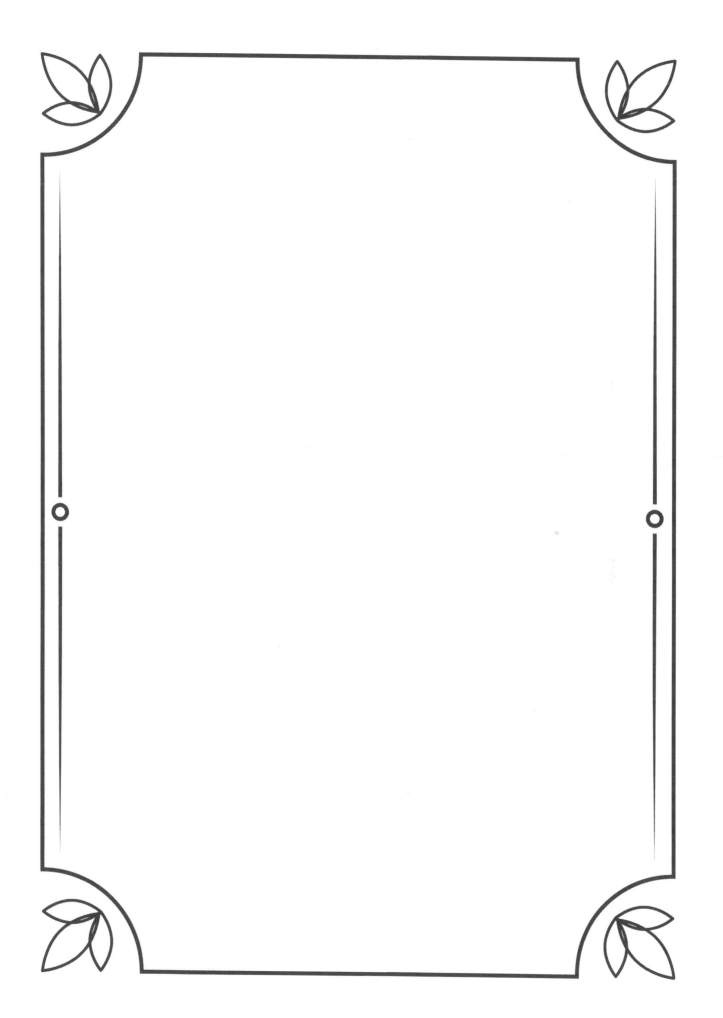

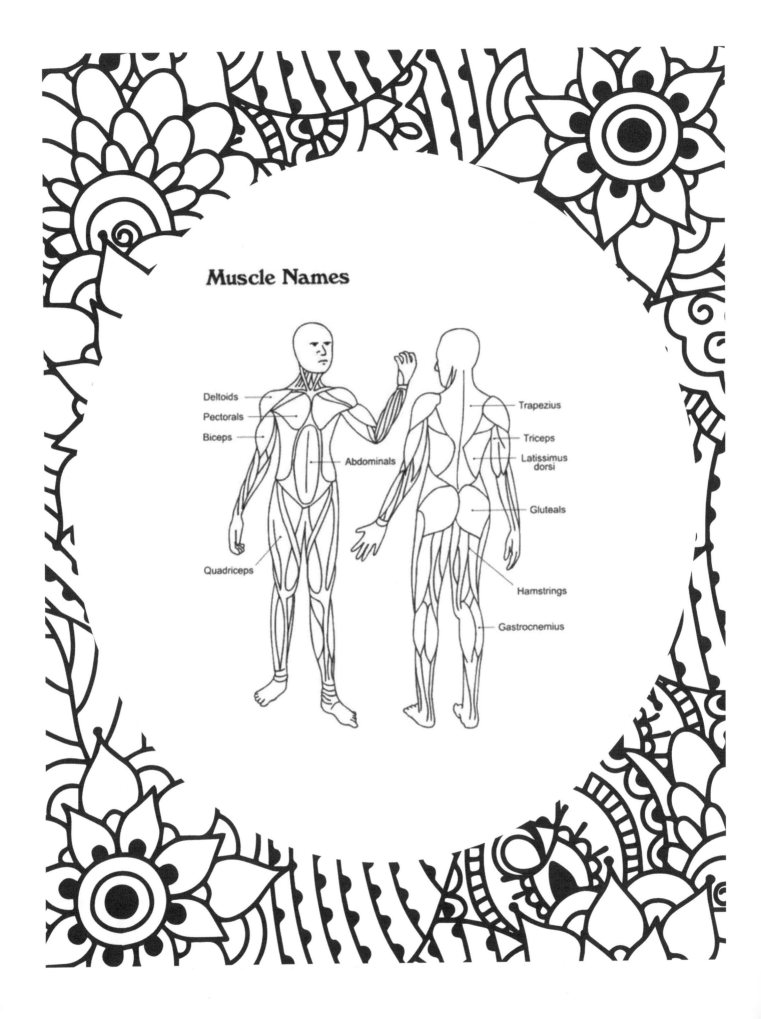

Muscle Names

Deltoids

Pectorals

Biceps

Abdominals

Quadriceps

Trapezius

Triceps

Latissimus dorsi

Gluteals

Hamstrings

Gastrocnemius

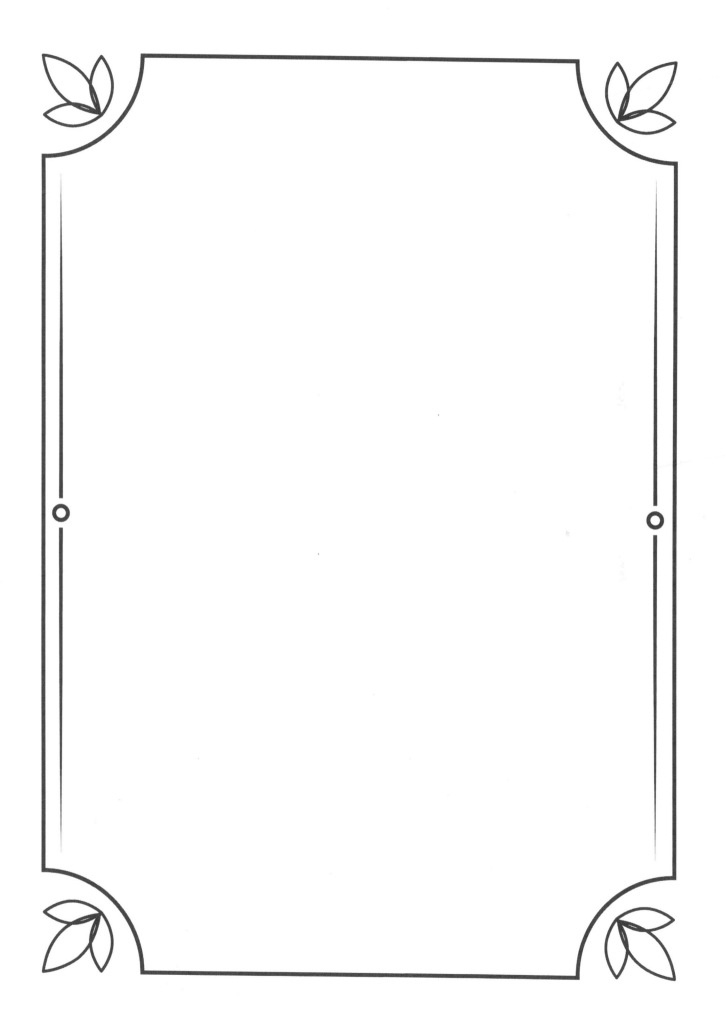

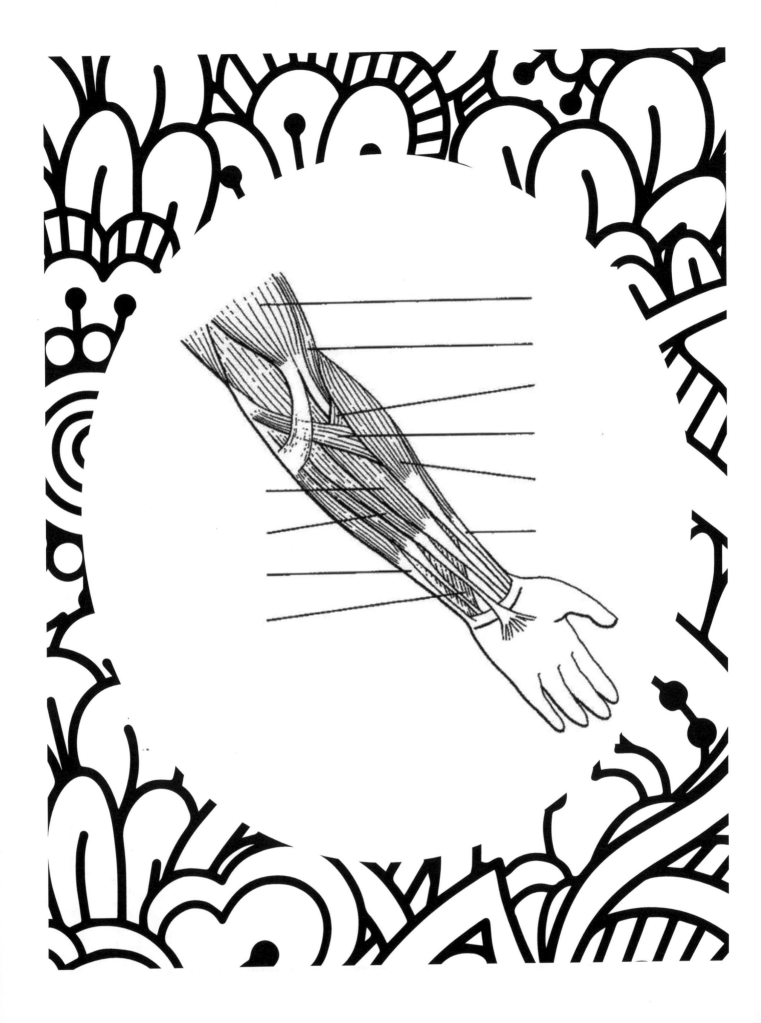

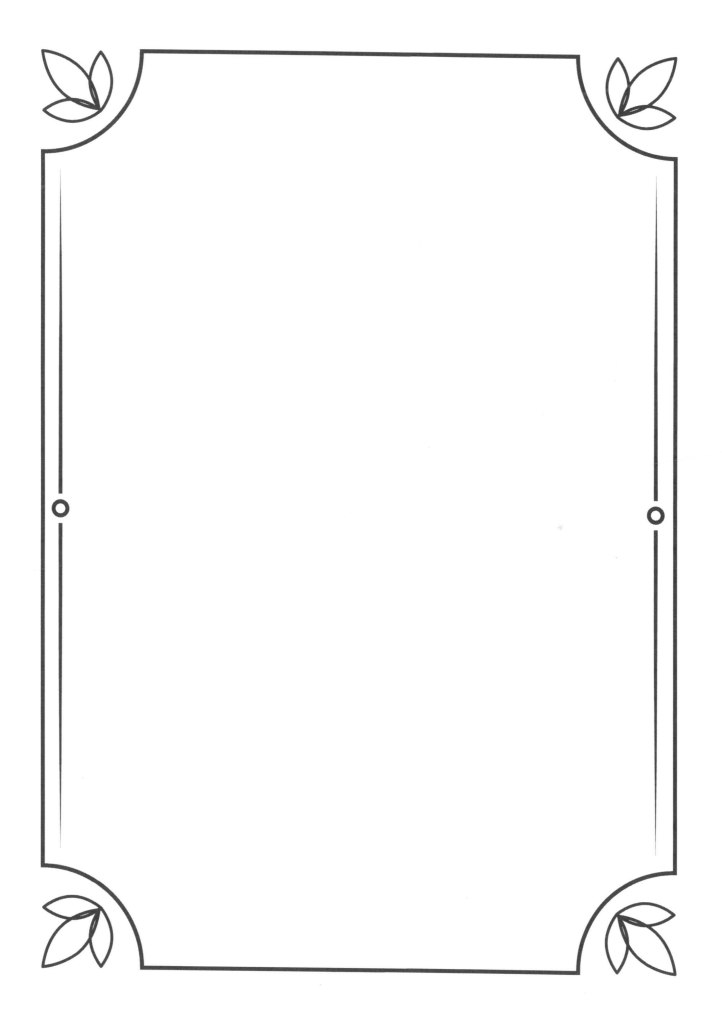

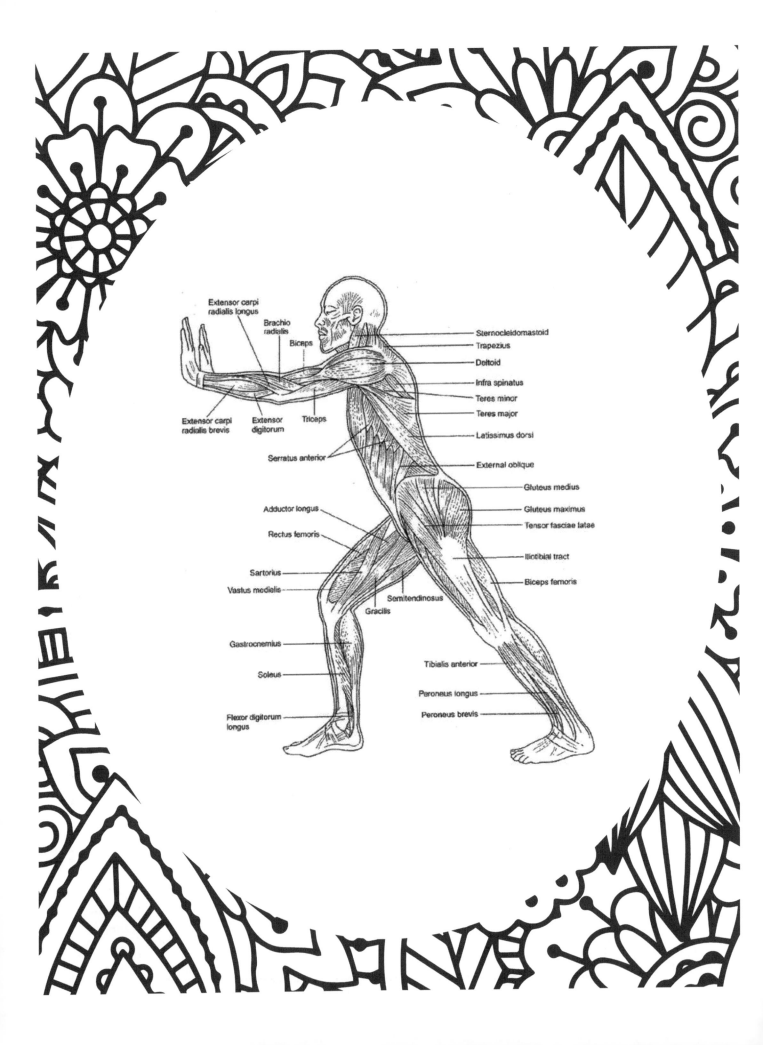

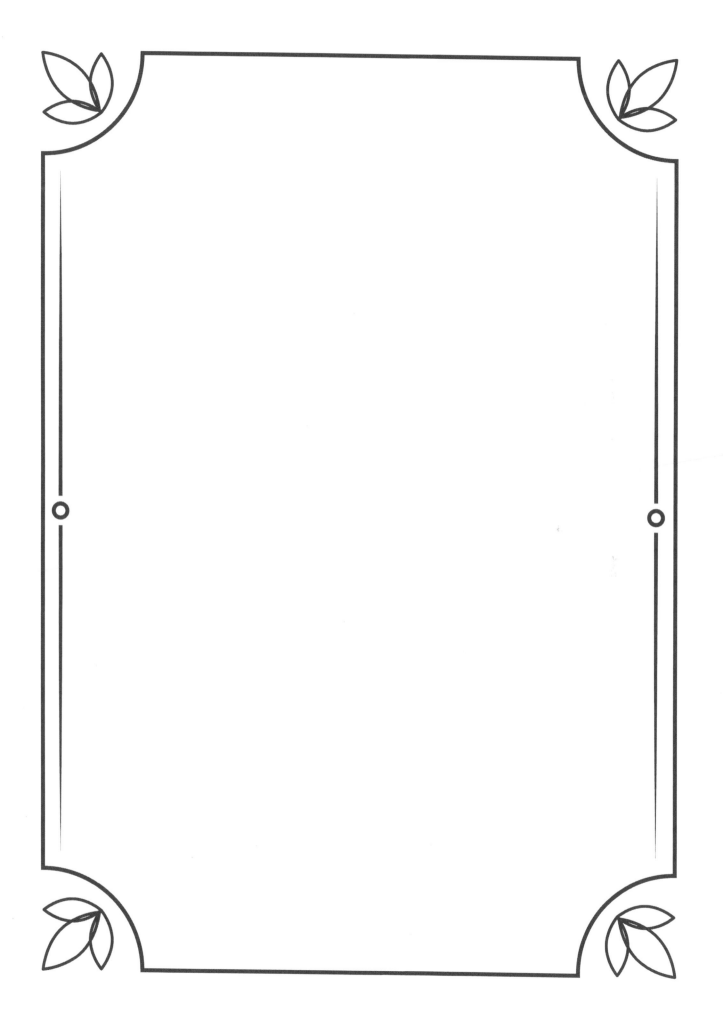

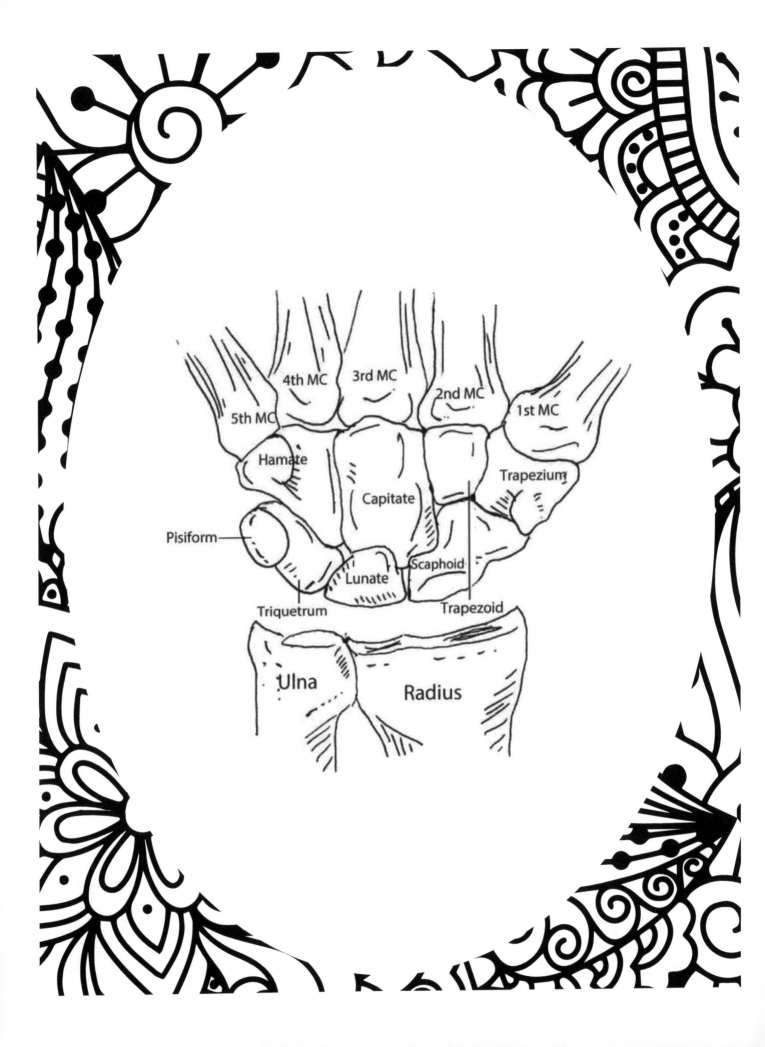

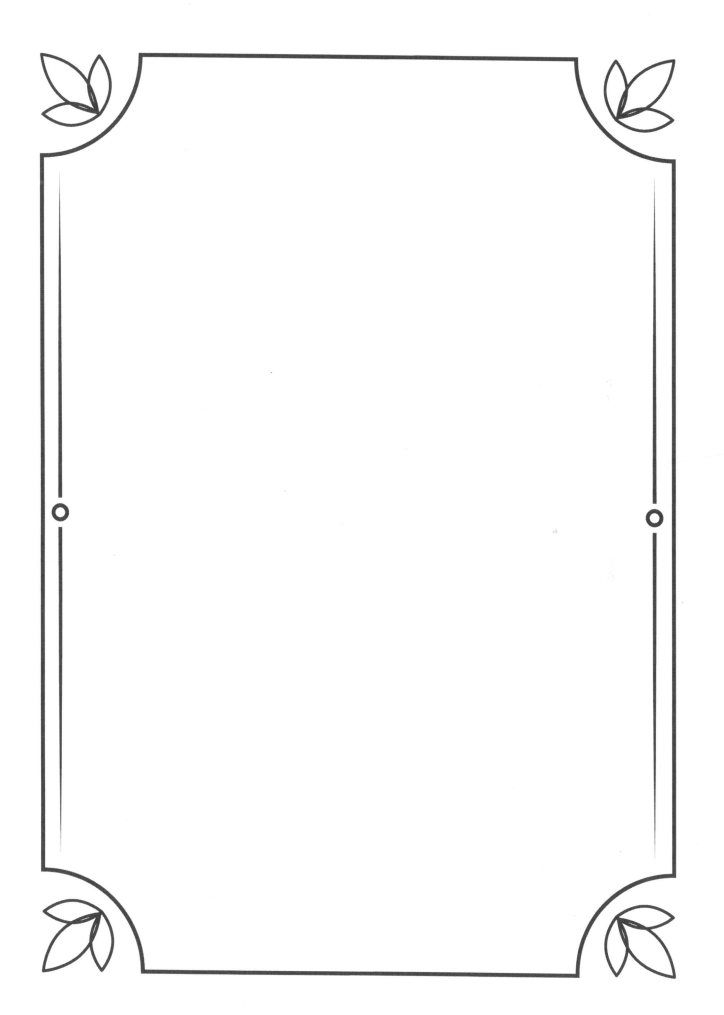

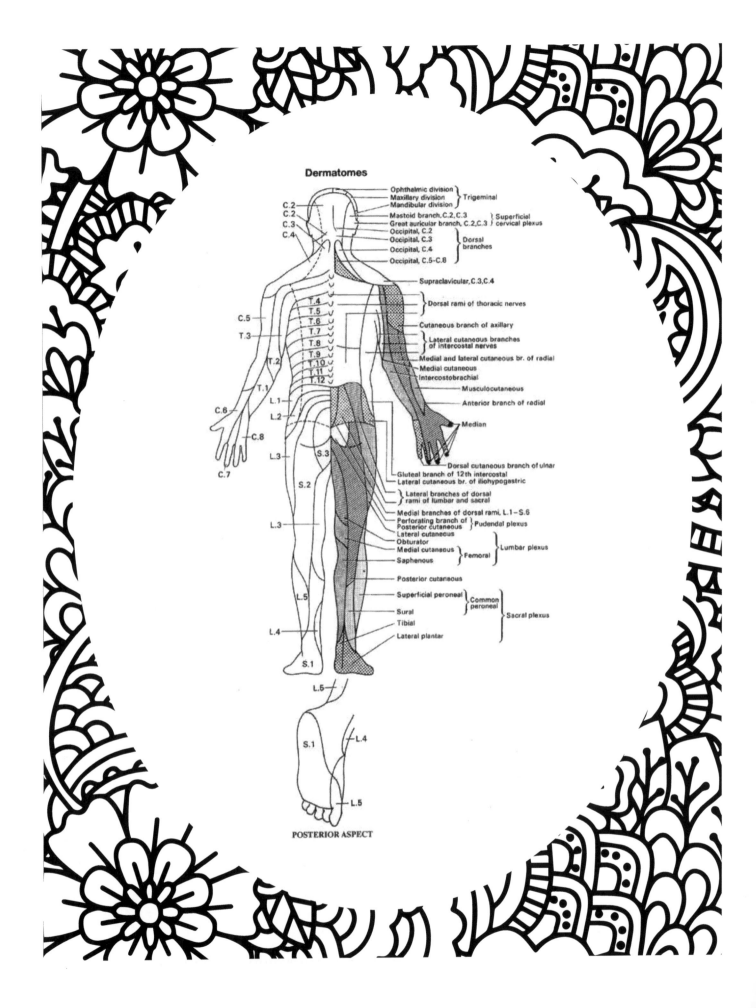

Dermatomes

Ophthalmic division ⎫
Maxillary division ⎬ Trigeminal
Mandibular division ⎭
C.2
C.2
C.3
C.4
Mastoid branch,C.2,C.3 ⎫ Superficial
Great auricular branch, C.2,C.3 ⎬ cervical plexus
Occipital, C.2
Occipital, C.3 ⎫ Dorsal
Occipital, C.4 ⎬ branches
Occipital, C.5-C.8

Supraclavicular,C.3,C.4

C.5
T.3
T.2
T.1
C.6
C.8
C.7

T.4
T.5
T.6
T.7
T.8
T.9
T.10
T.11
T.12
L.1
L.2
L.3

S.3
S.2
L.3
L.5
L.4
S.1

Dorsal rami of thoracic nerves
Cutaneous branch of axillary
Lateral cutaneous branches
of intercostal nerves
Medial and lateral cutaneous br. of radial
Medial cutaneous
Intercostobrachial
Musculocutaneous
Anterior branch of radial
Median

Dorsal cutaneous branch of ulnar
Gluteal branch of 12th intercostal
Lateral cutaneous br. of iliohypogastric
Lateral branches of dorsal
rami of lumbar and sacral
Medial branches of dorsal rami, L.1–S.6
Perforating branch of
Posterior cutaneous ⎬ Pudendal plexus
Lateral cutaneous
Obturator
Medial cutaneous ⎫ Femoral ⎫ Lumbar plexus
Saphenous ⎭
Posterior cutaneous
Superficial peroneal ⎫ Common
peroneal
Sural
Tibial ⎬ Sacral plexus
Lateral plantar

L.5

S.1   L.4
             L.5

POSTERIOR ASPECT

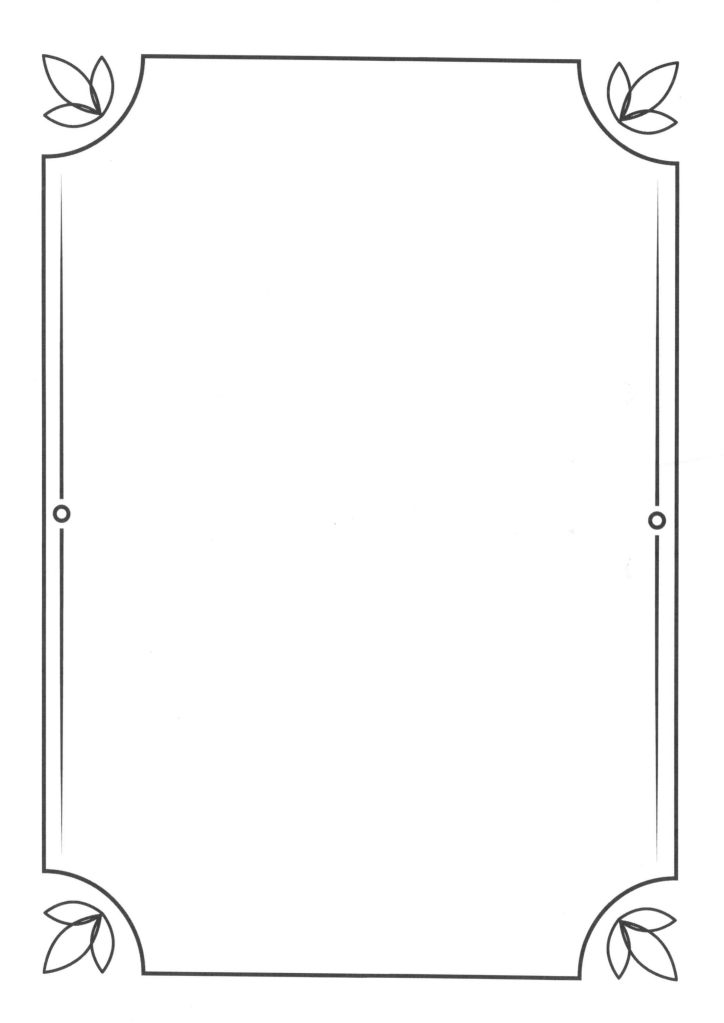

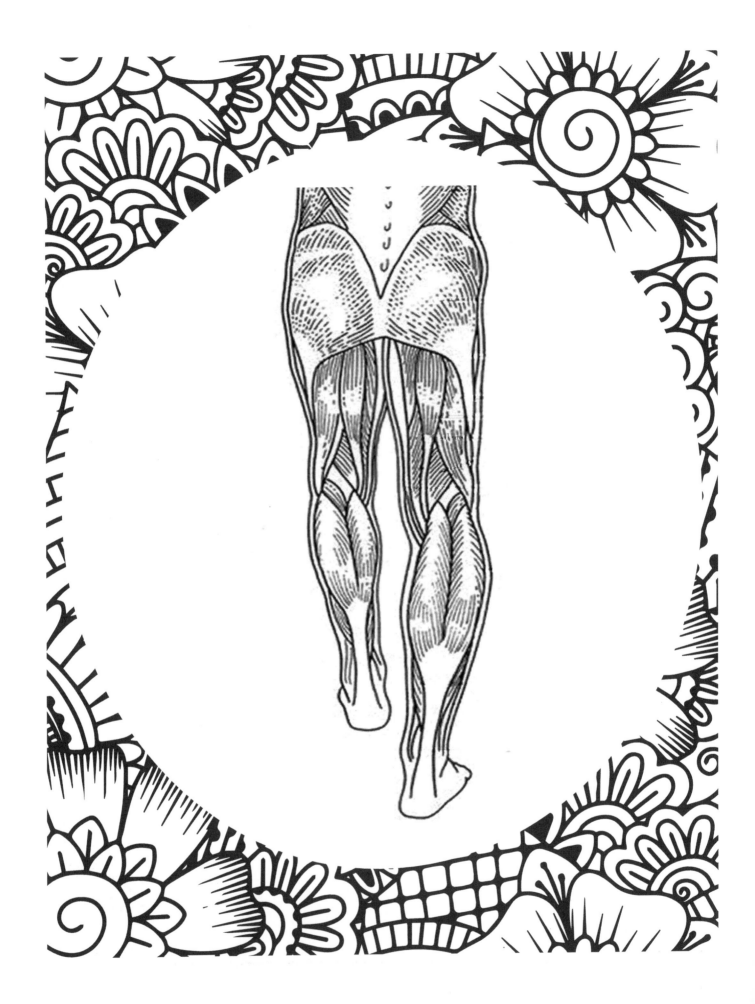

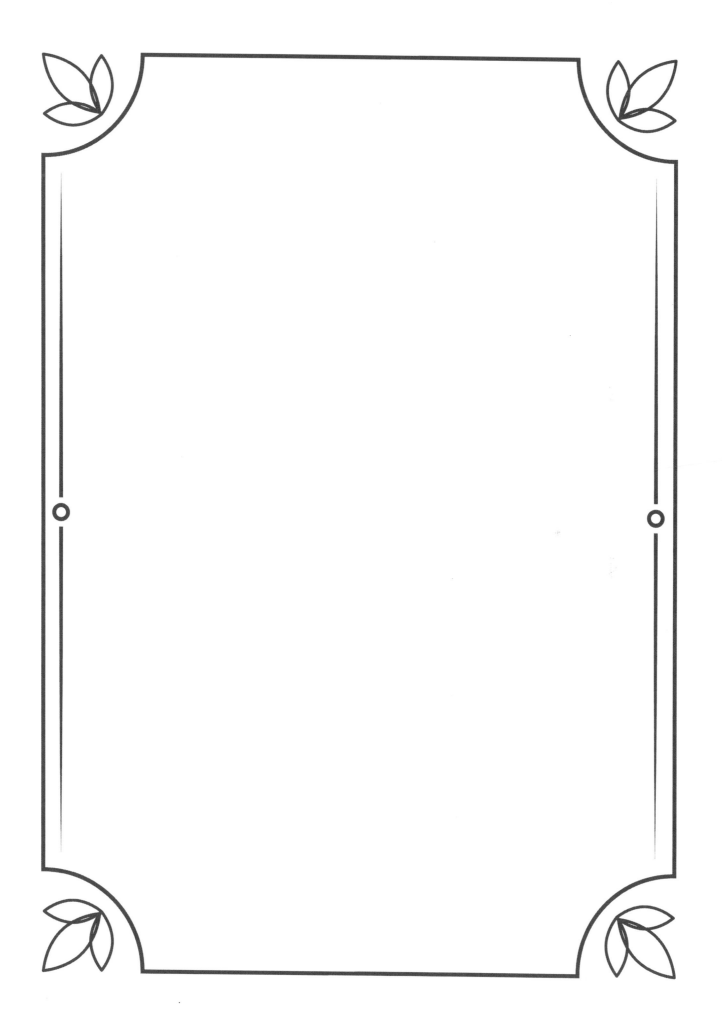

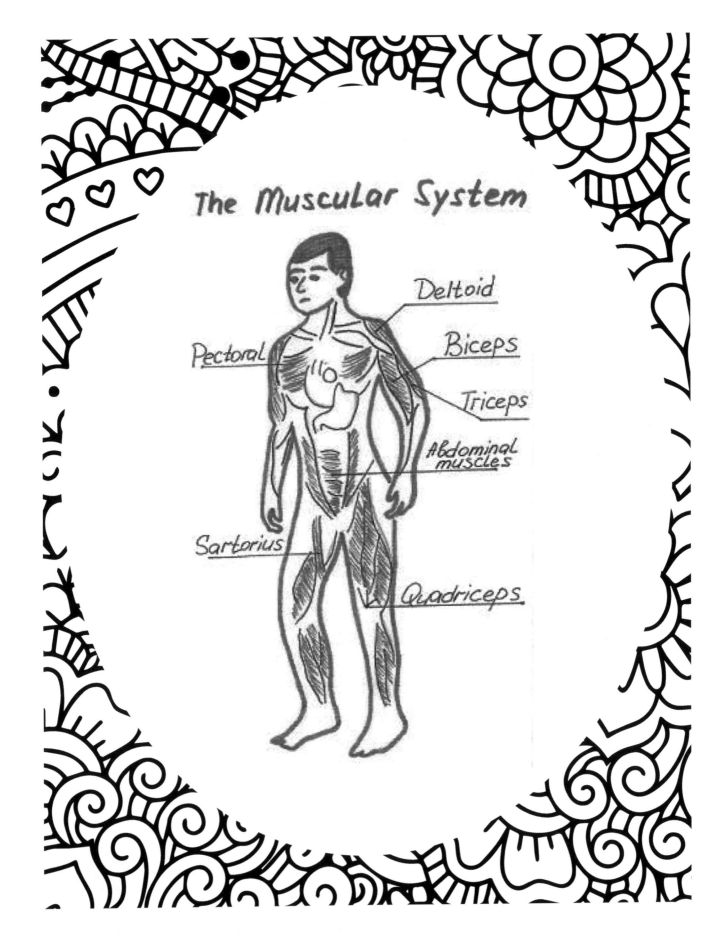

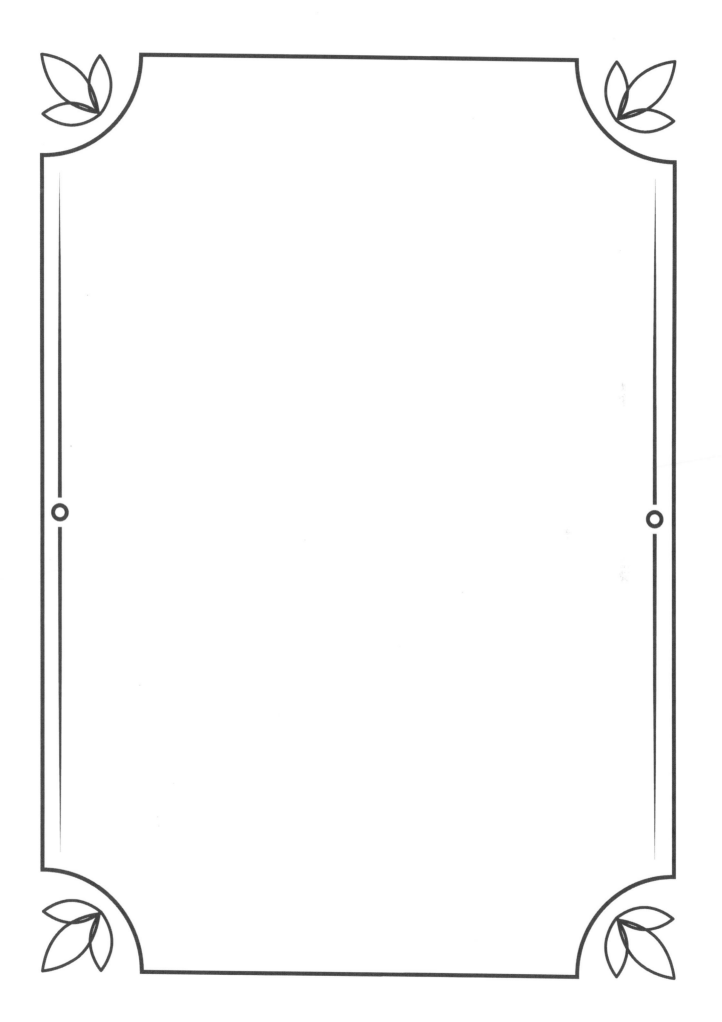

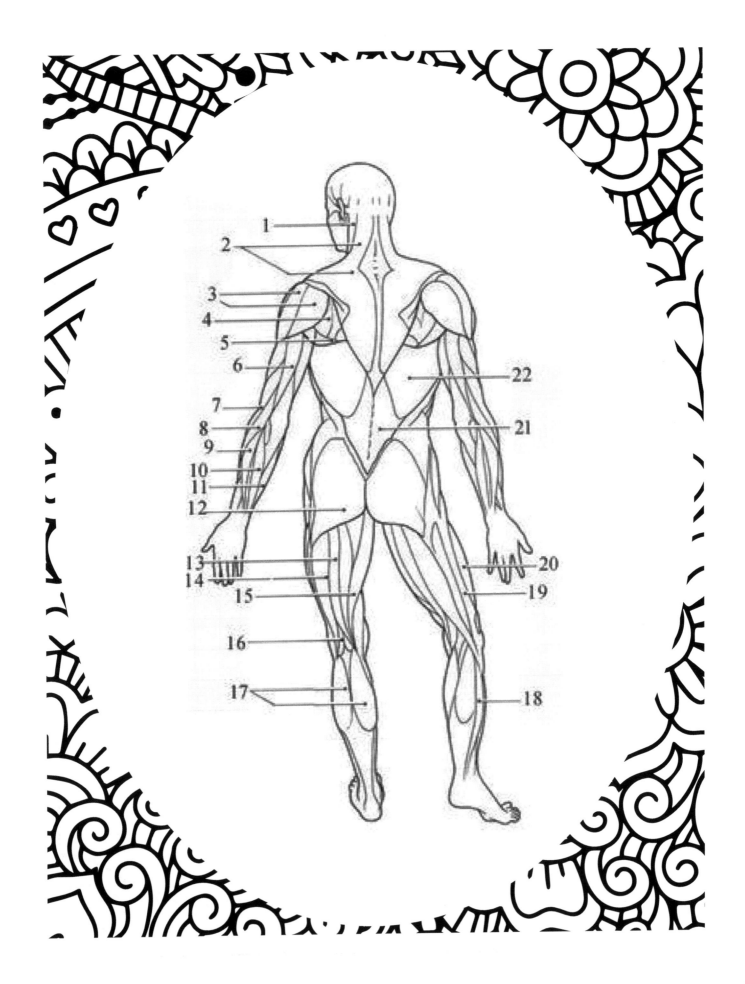

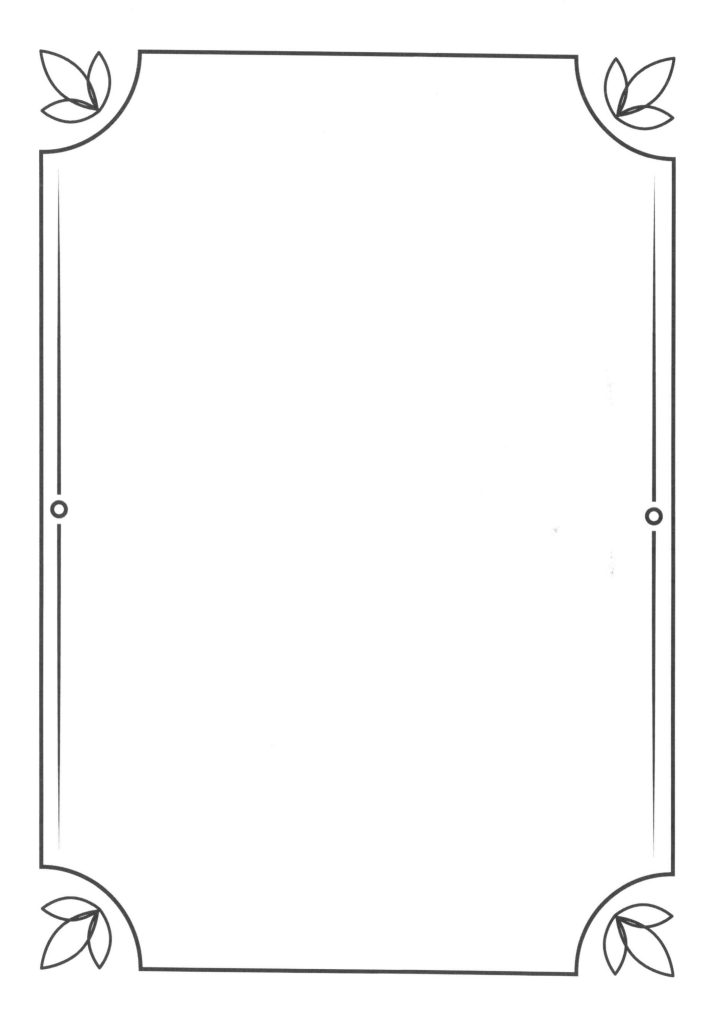

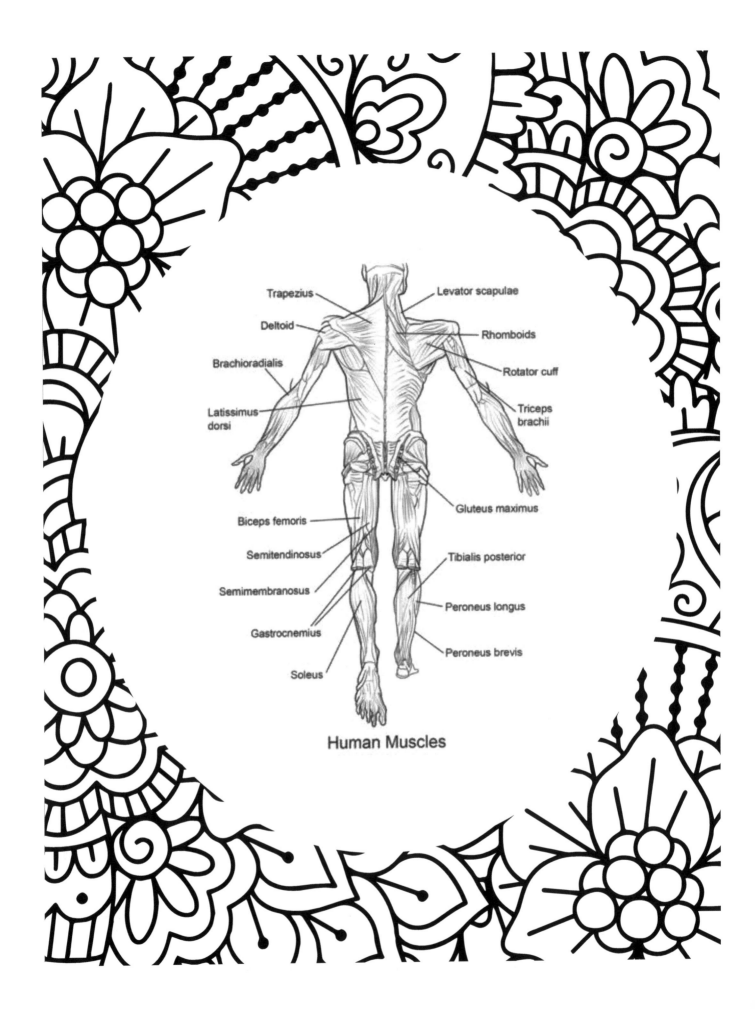

Trapezius

Levator scapulae

Deltoid

Rhomboids

Brachioradialis

Rotator cuff

Latissimus dorsi

Triceps brachii

Gluteus maximus

Biceps femoris

Semitendinosus

Tibialis posterior

Semimembranosus

Peroneus longus

Gastrocnemius

Peroneus brevis

Soleus

Human Muscles

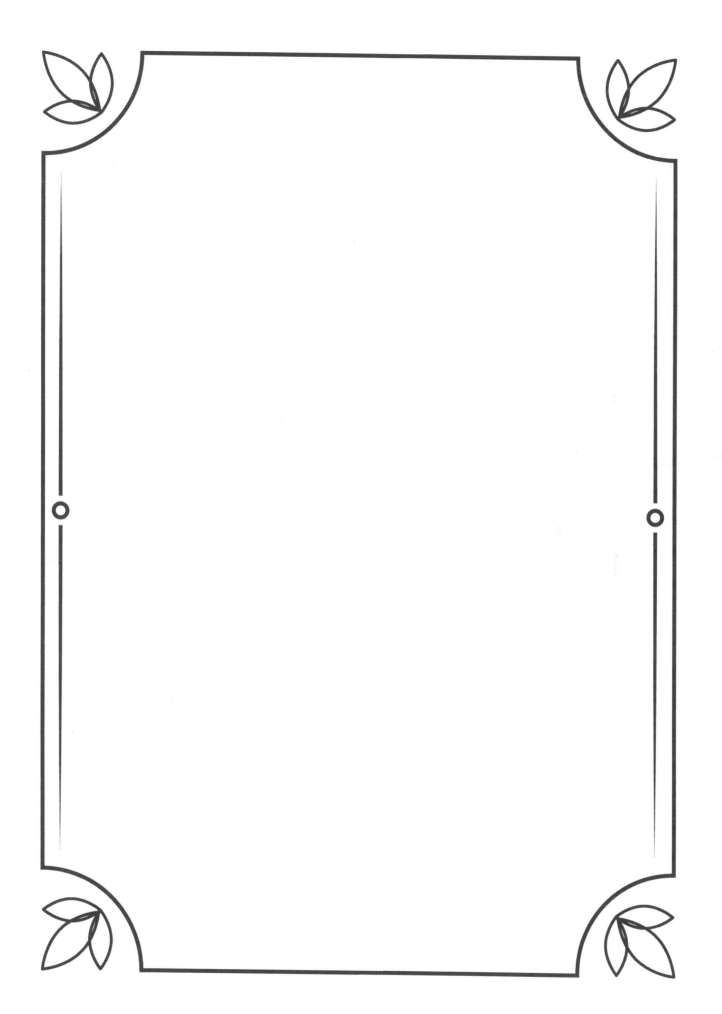

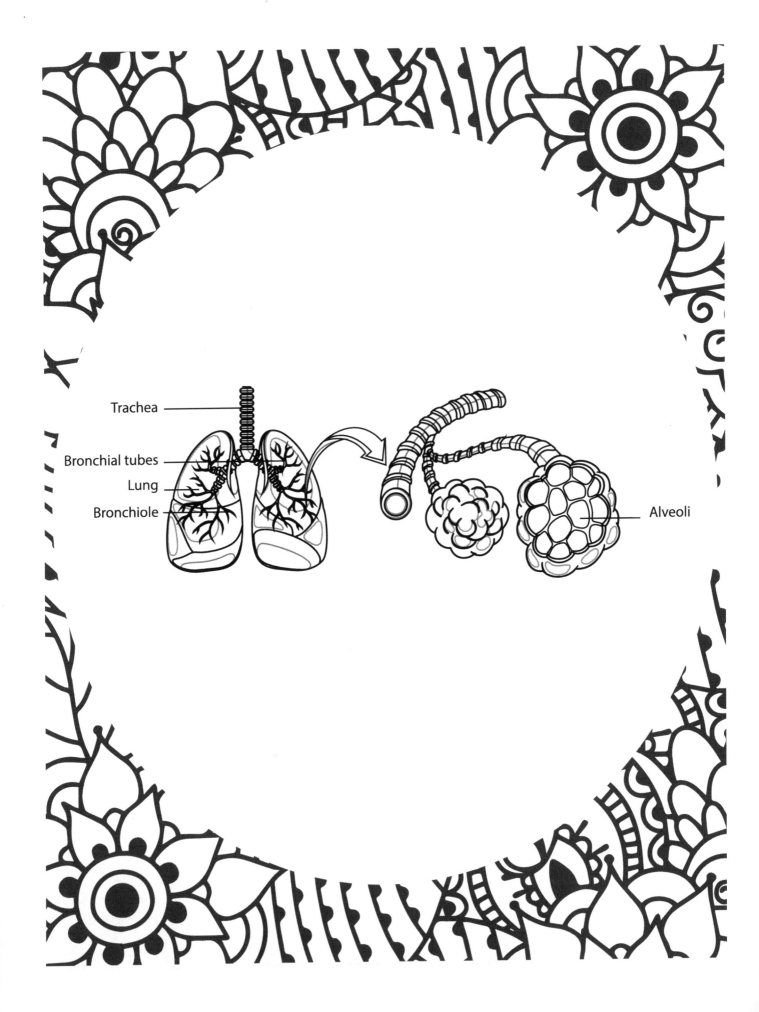

Trachea

Bronchial tubes

Lung

Bronchiole

Alveoli

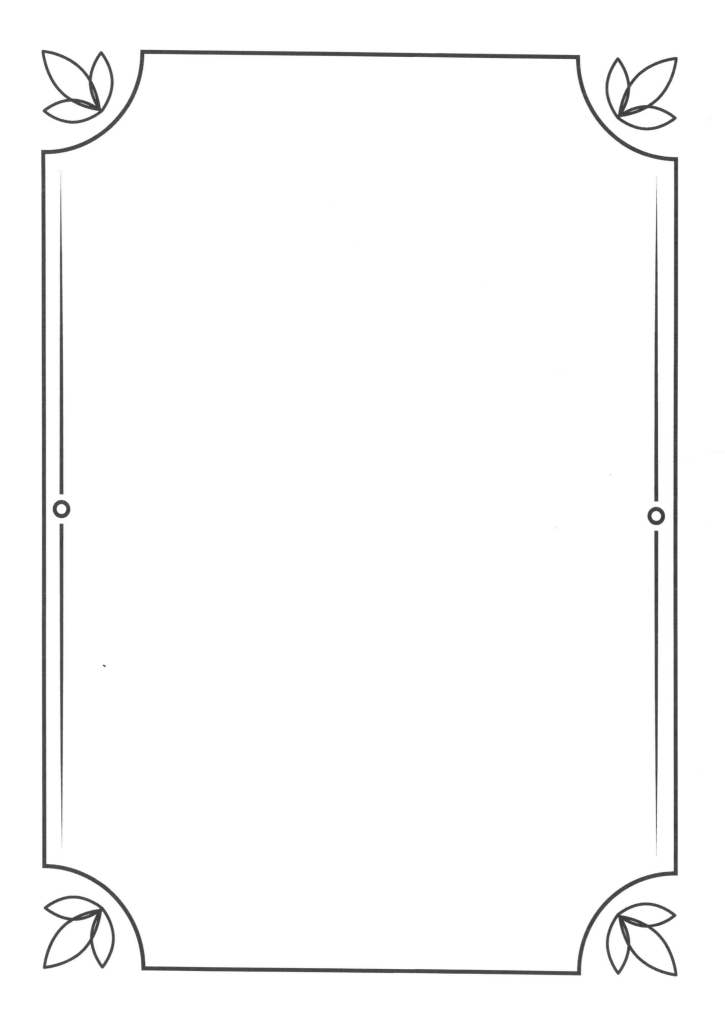

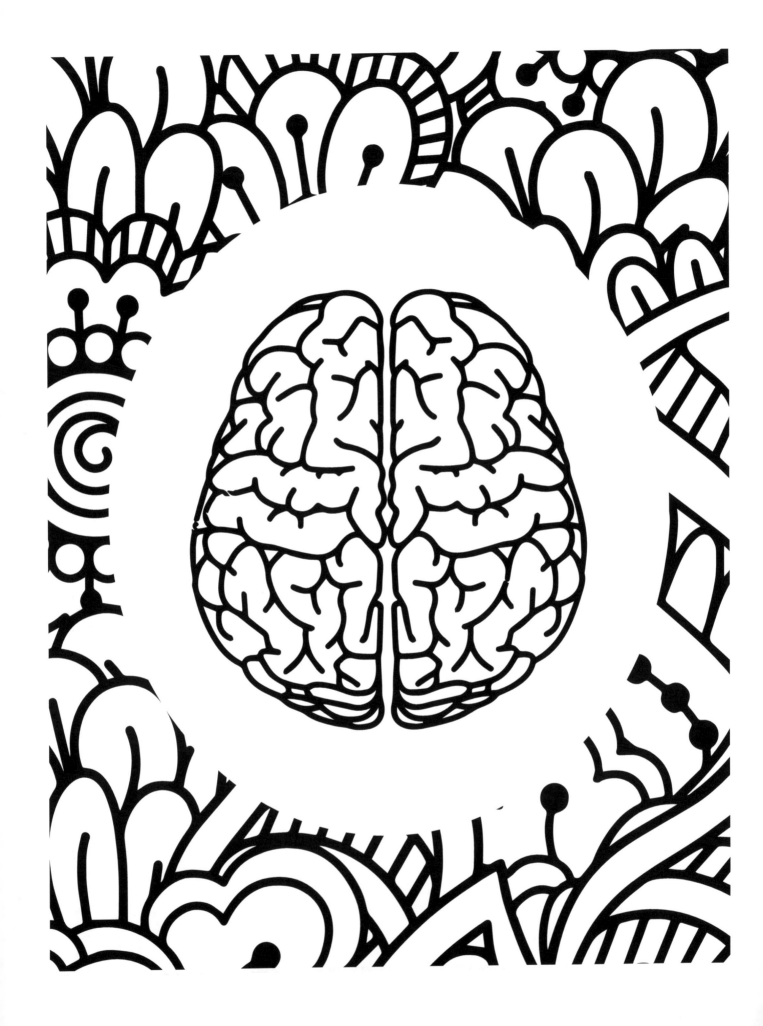

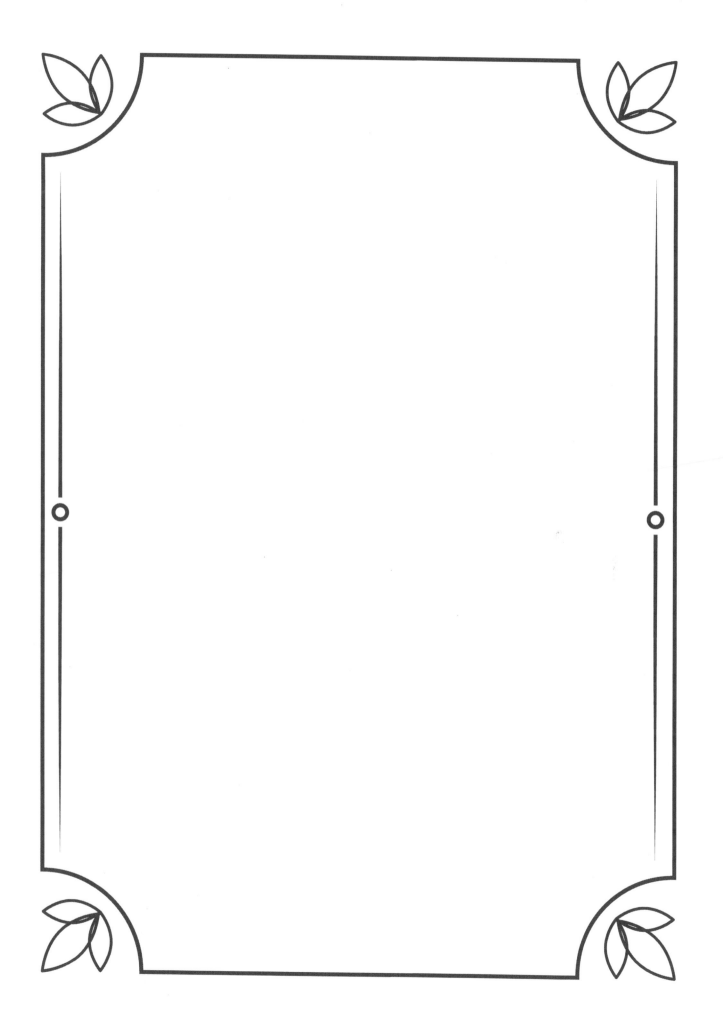

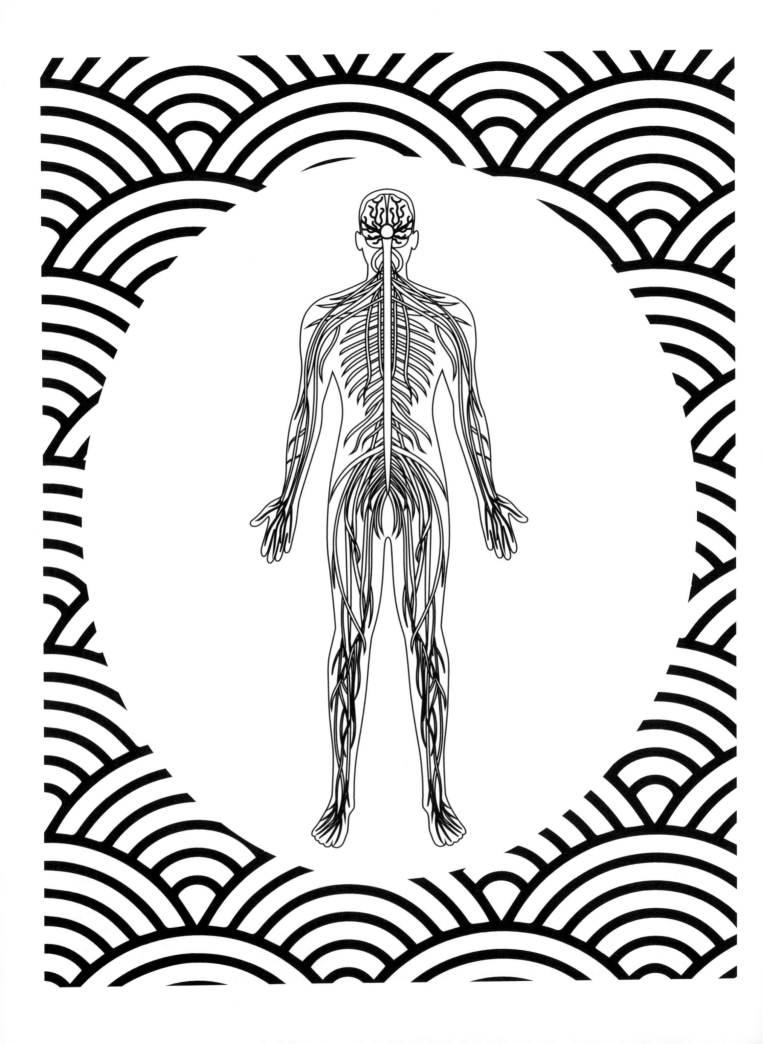

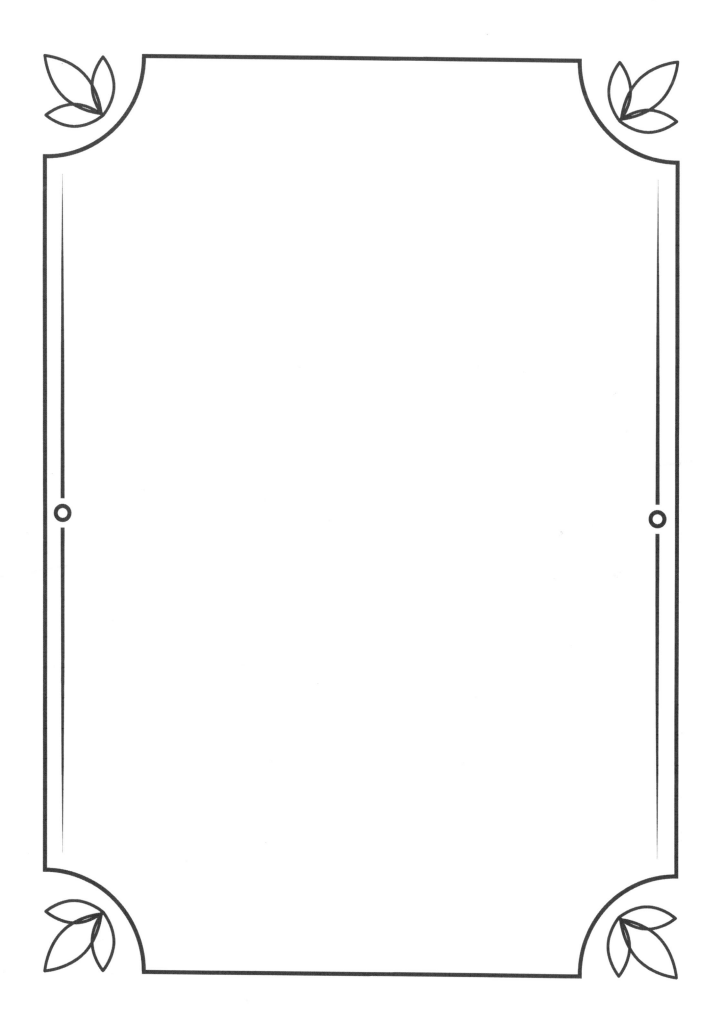

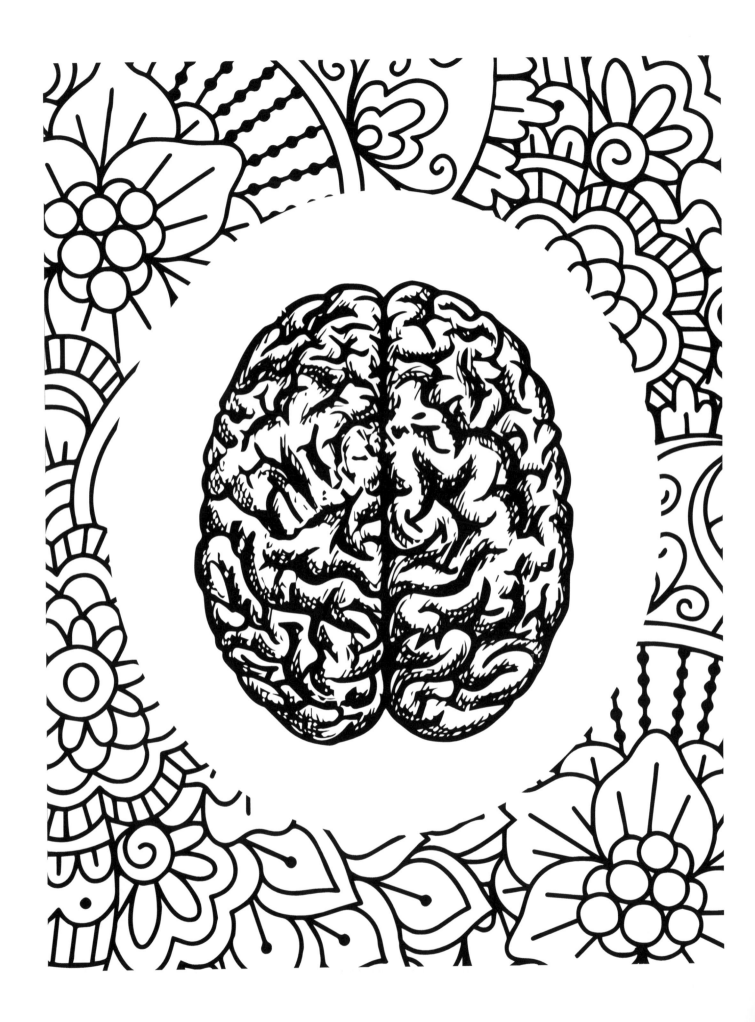

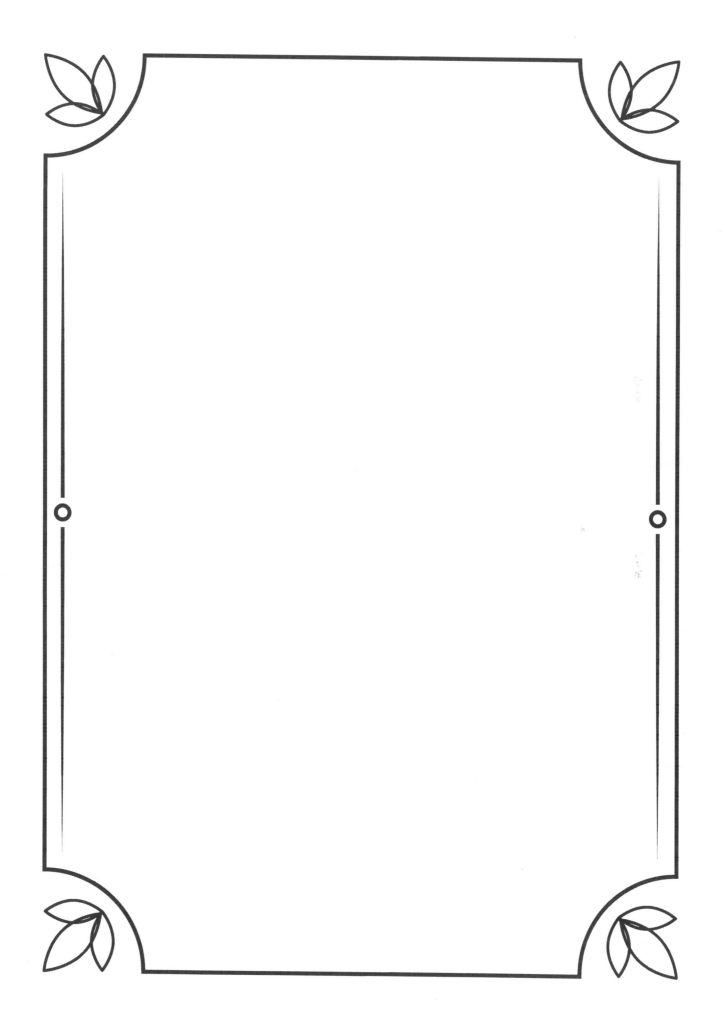

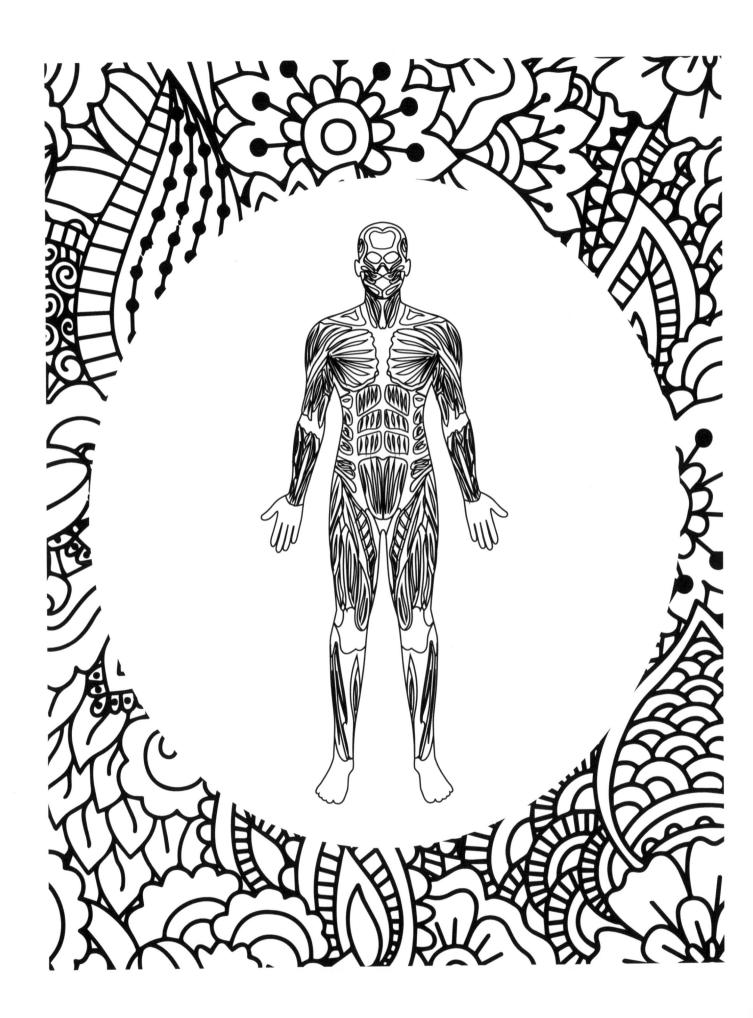

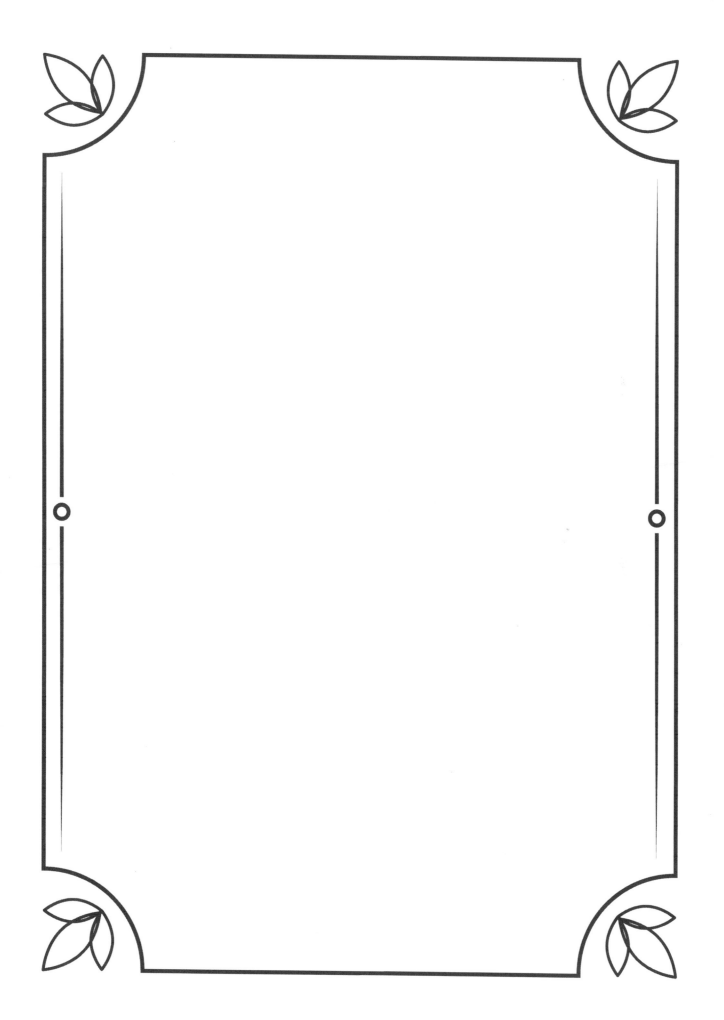

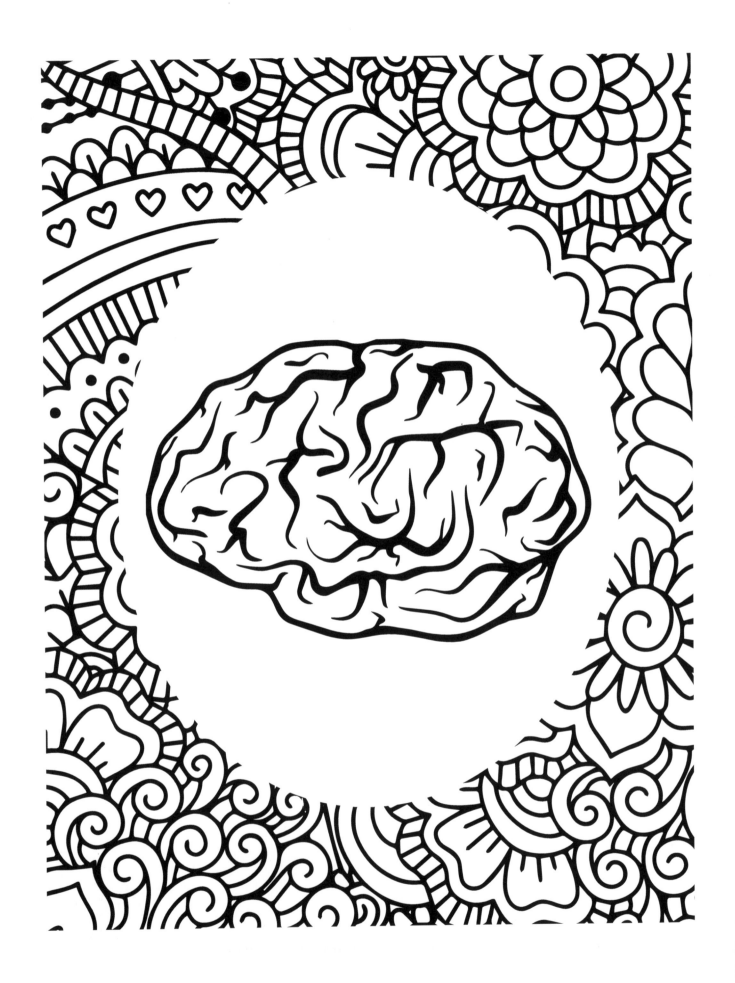

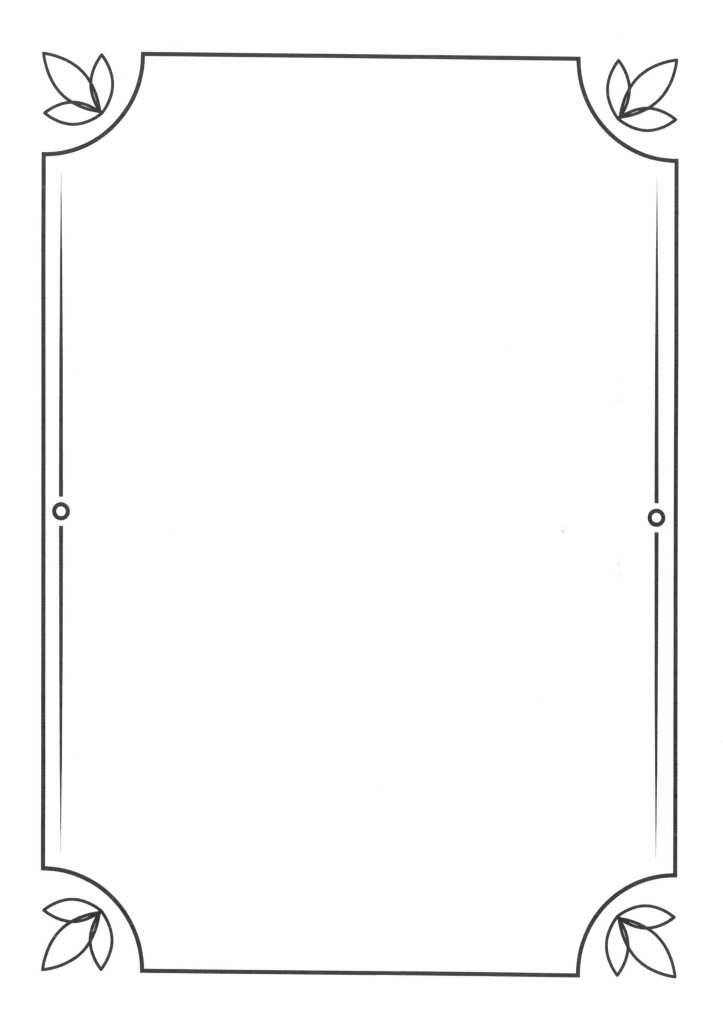

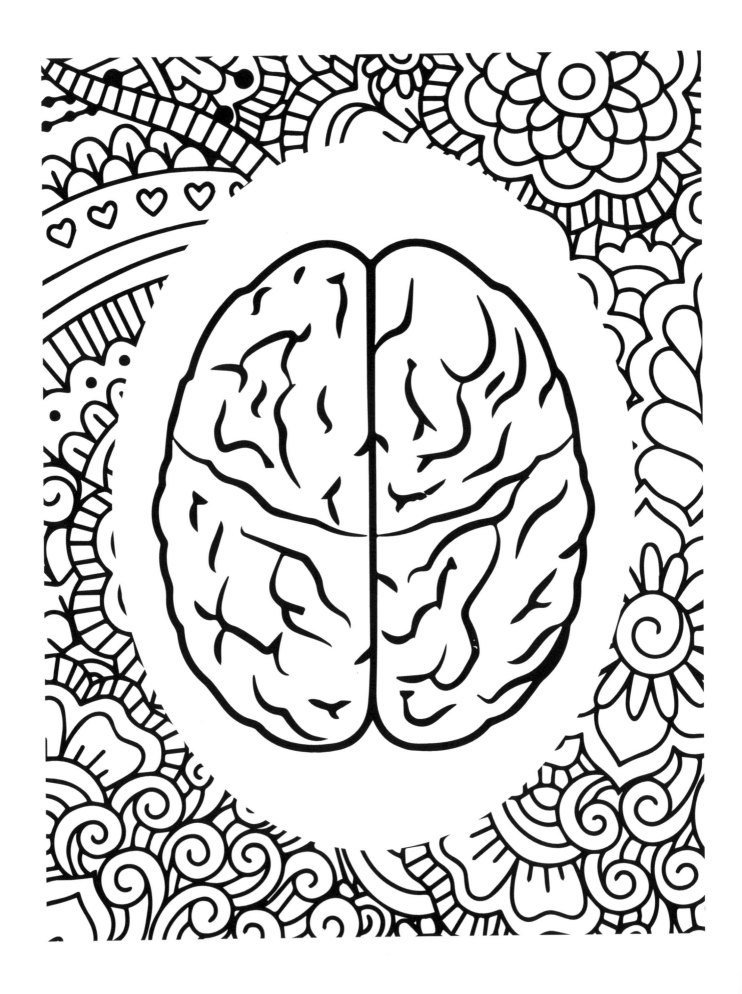

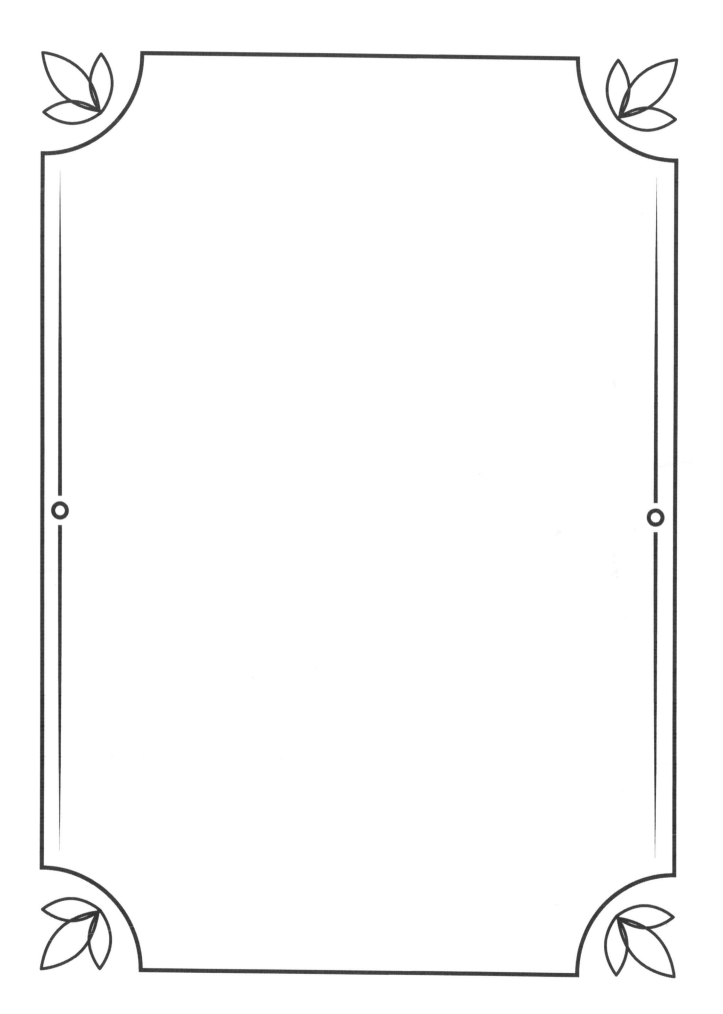

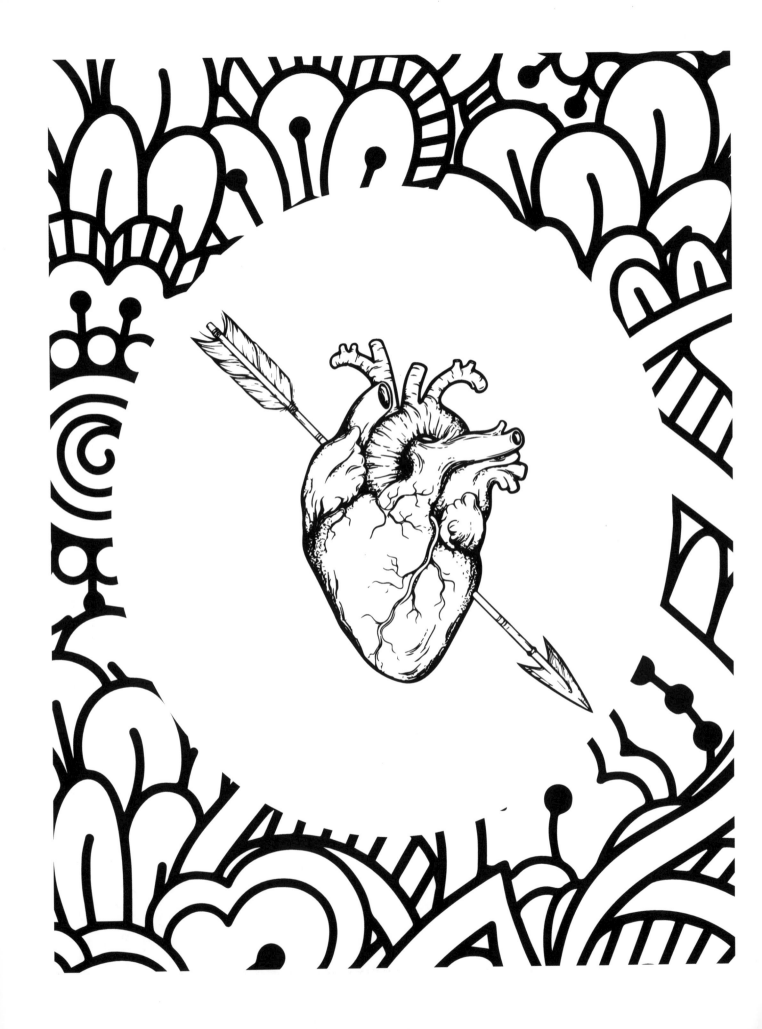

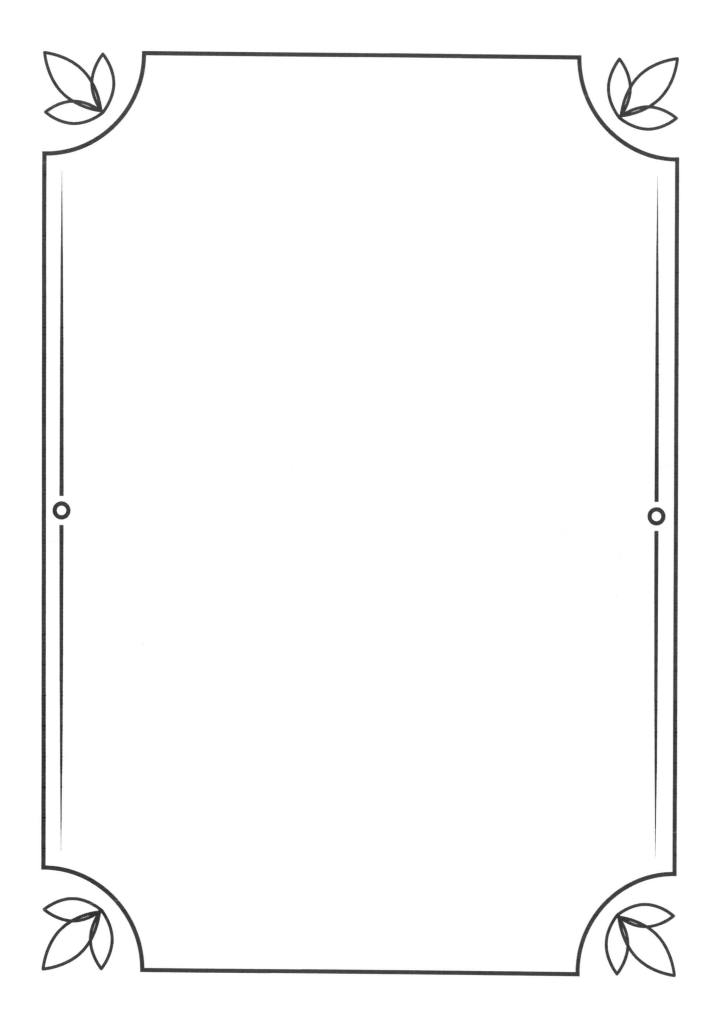

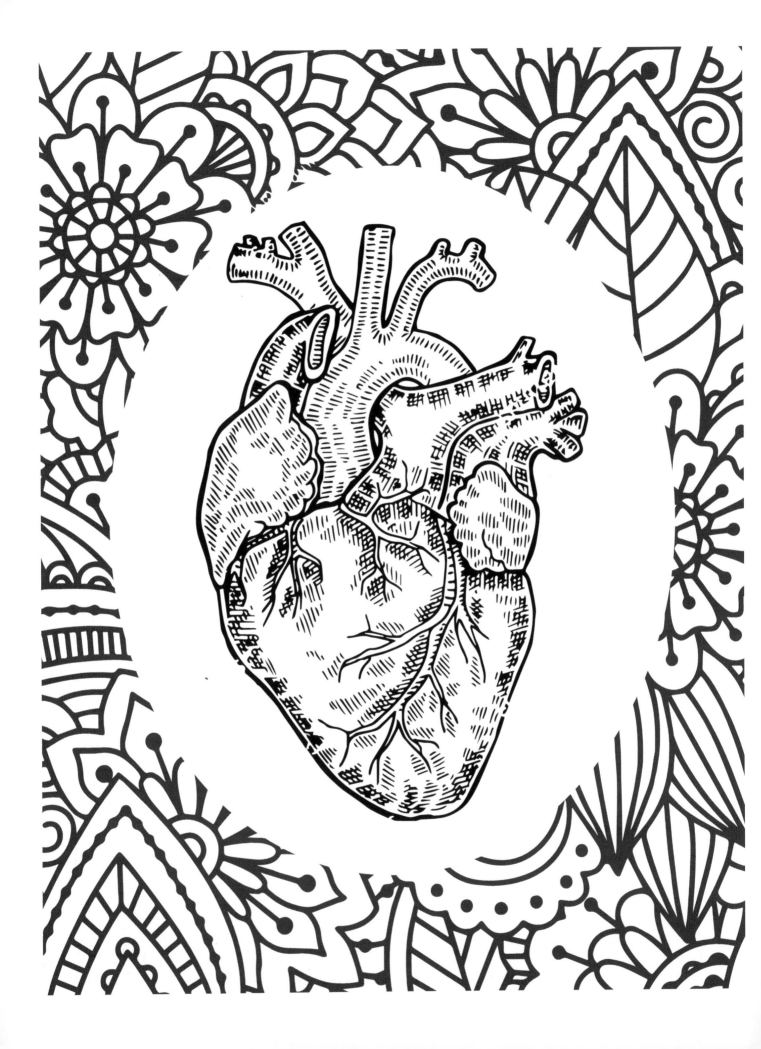

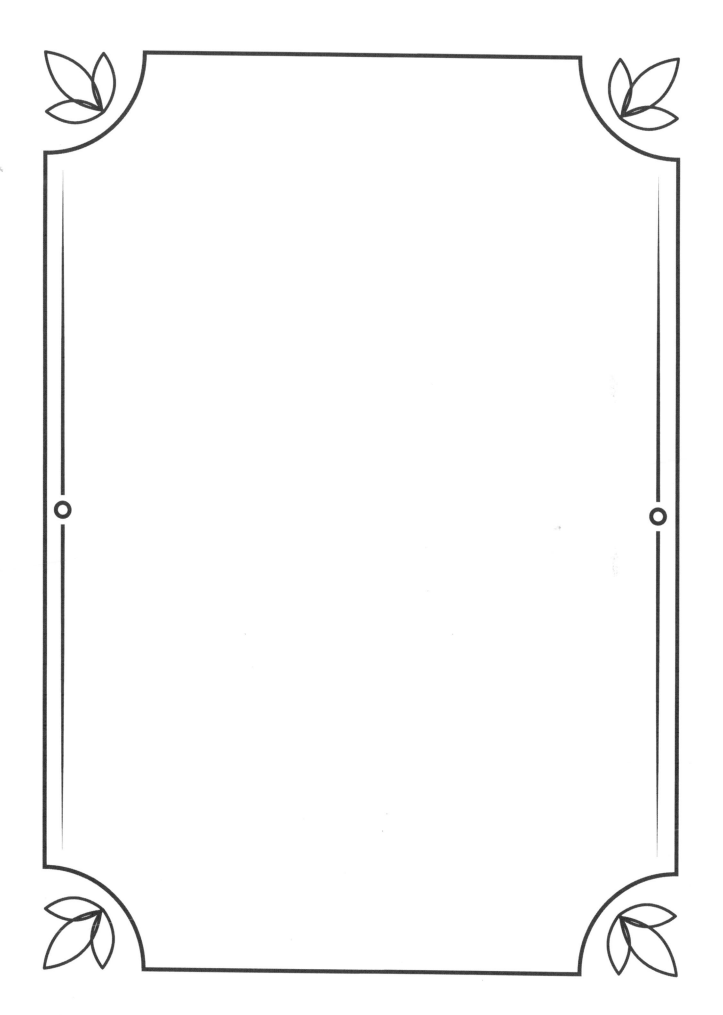

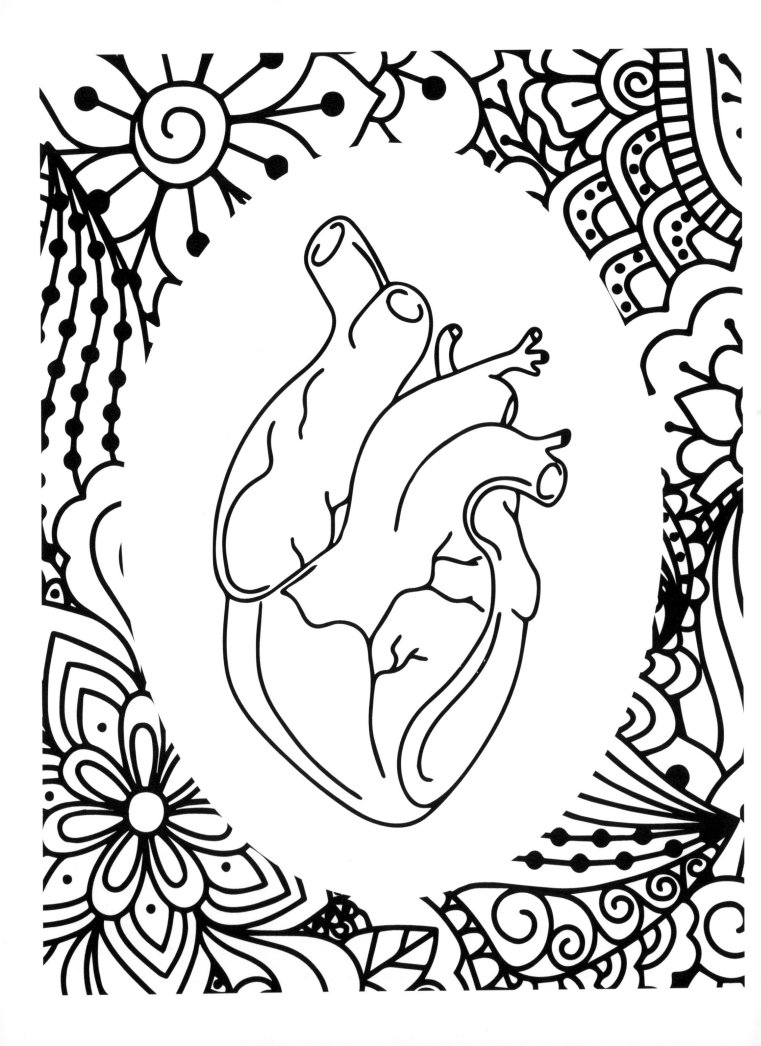

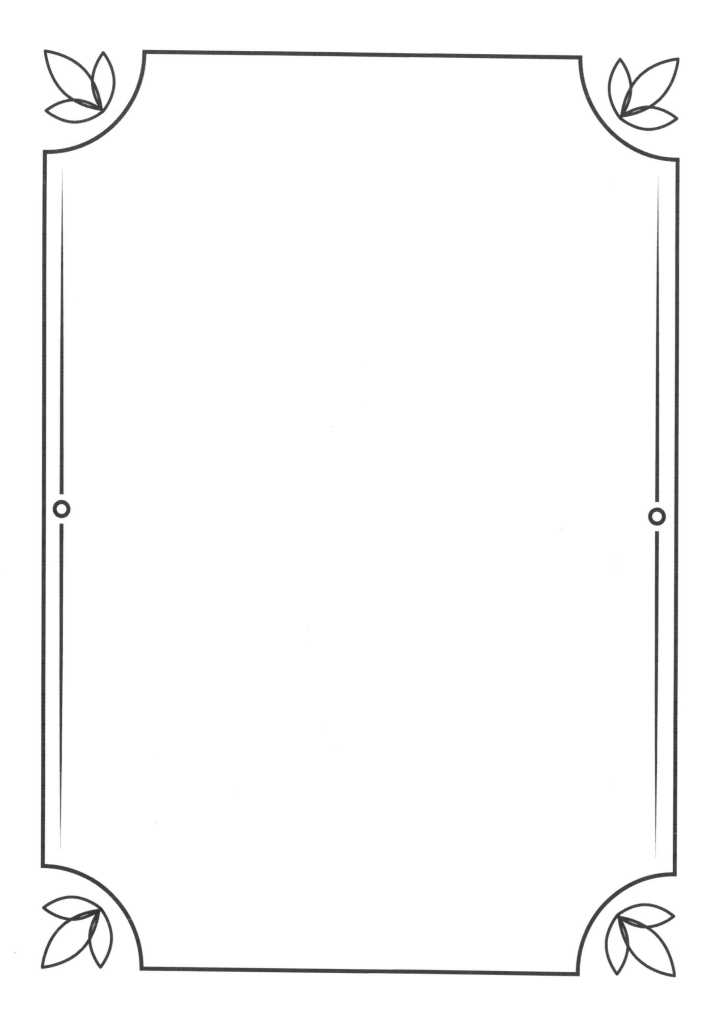

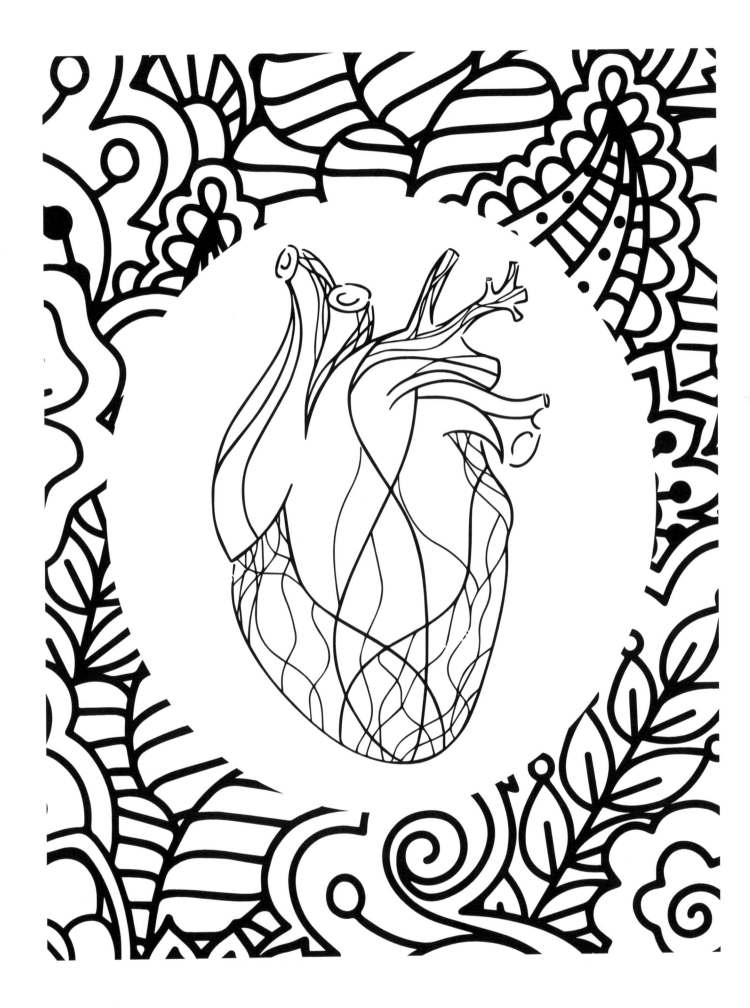

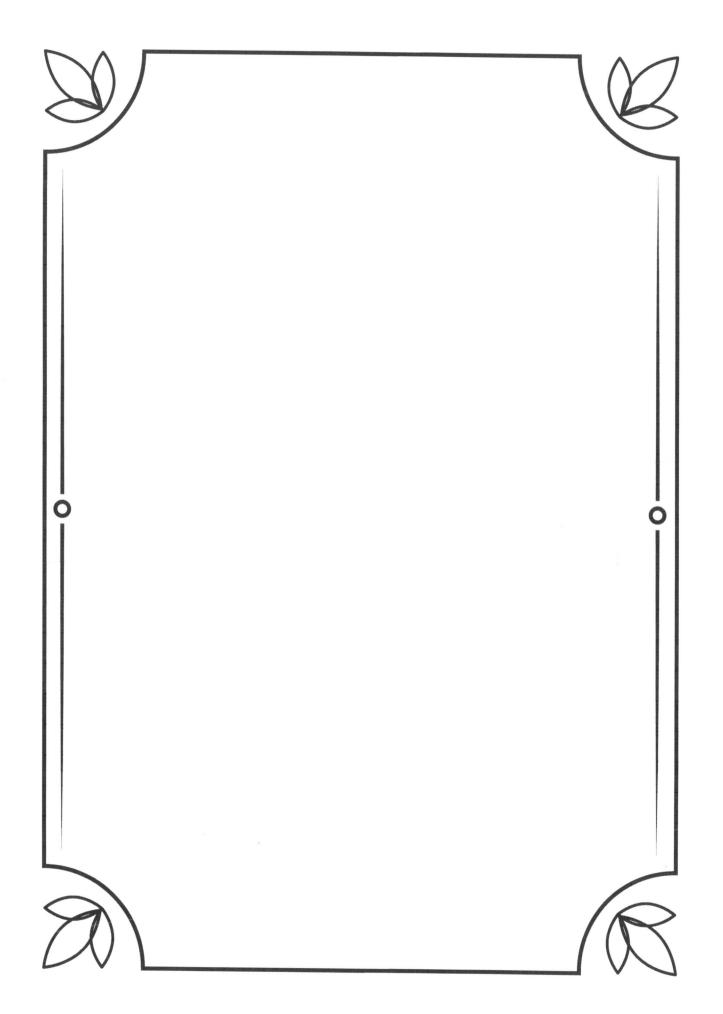

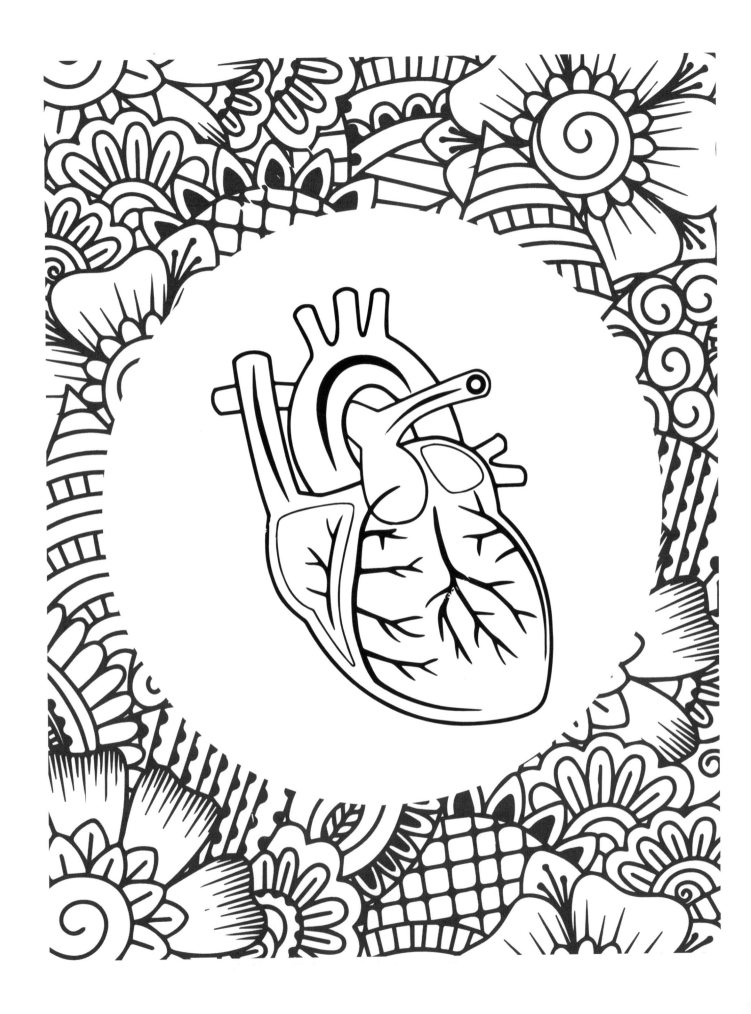

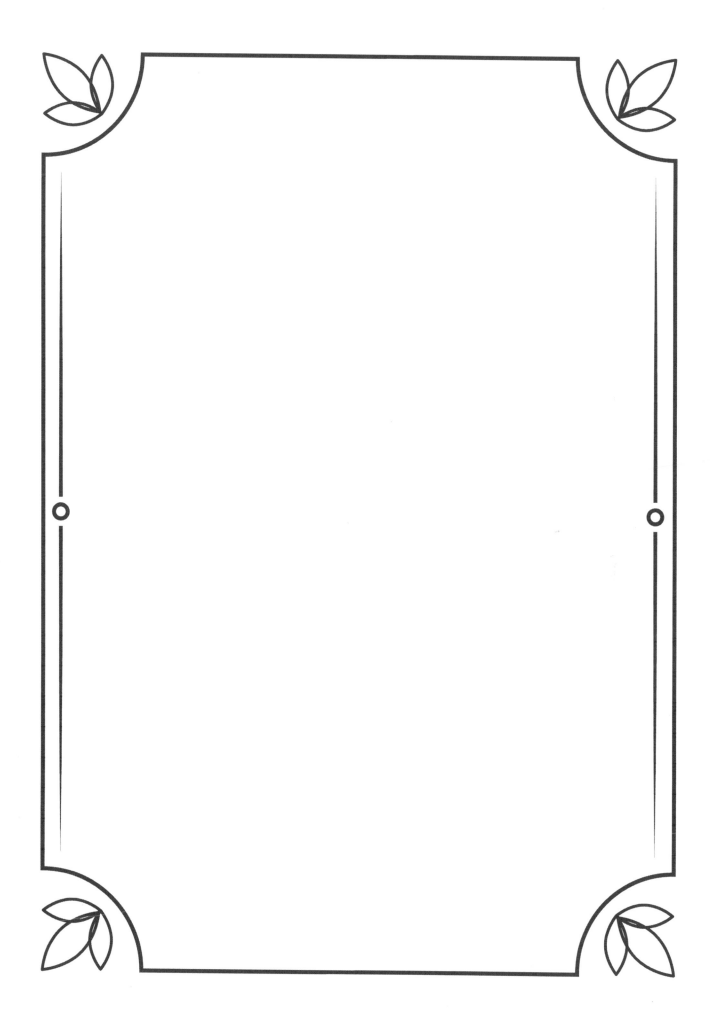

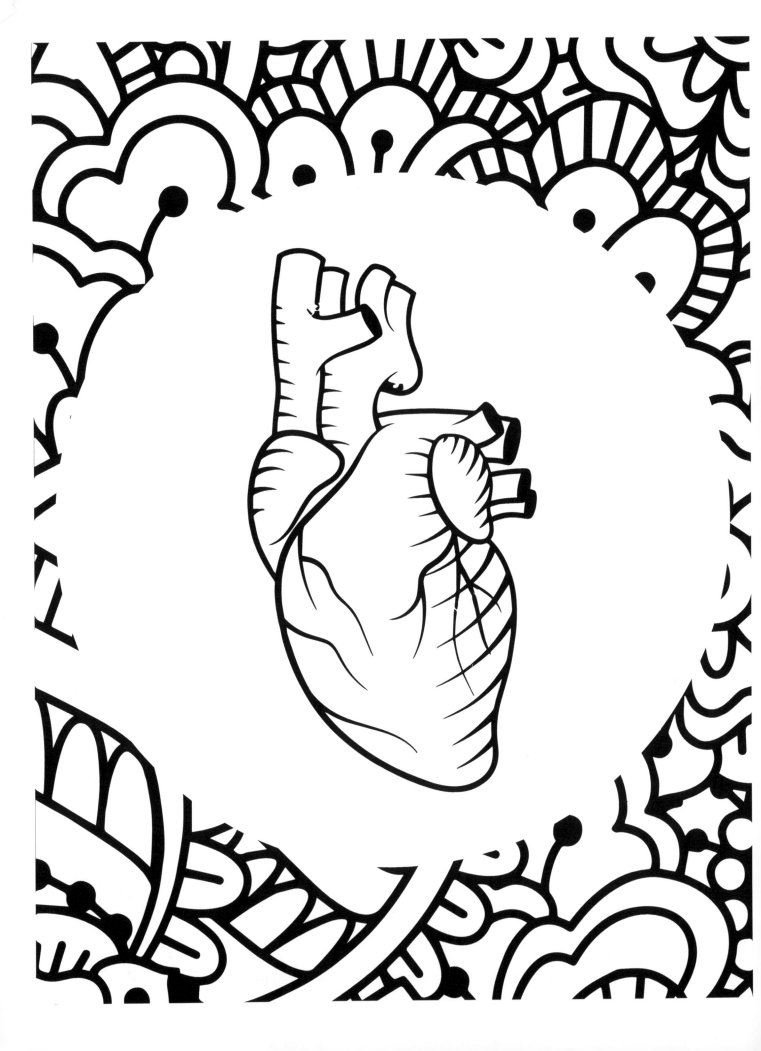

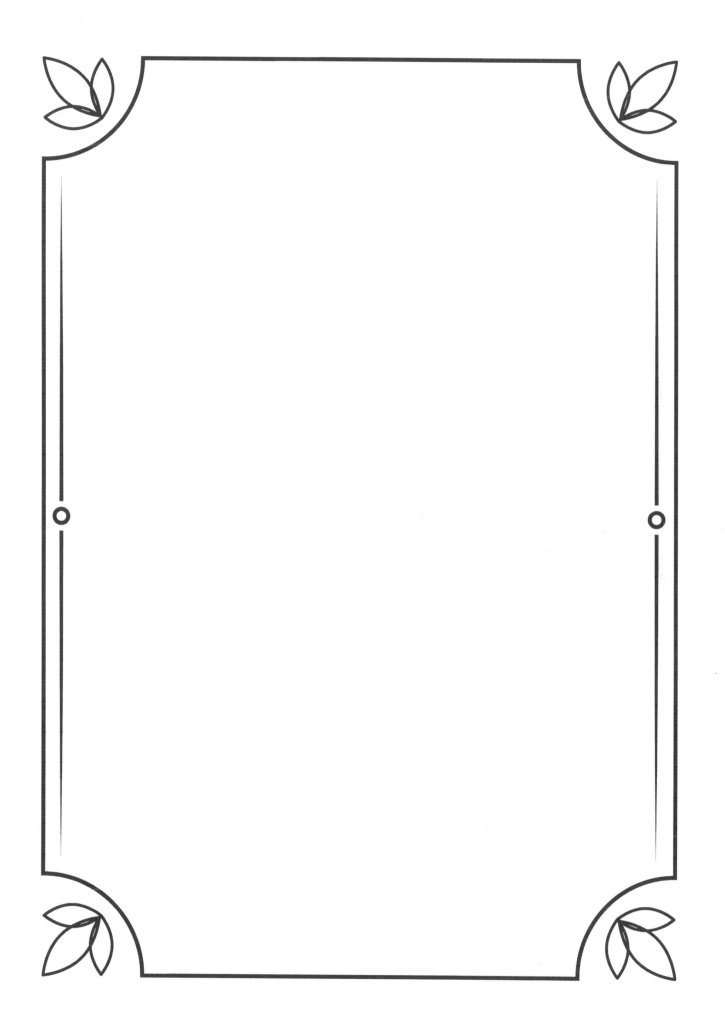

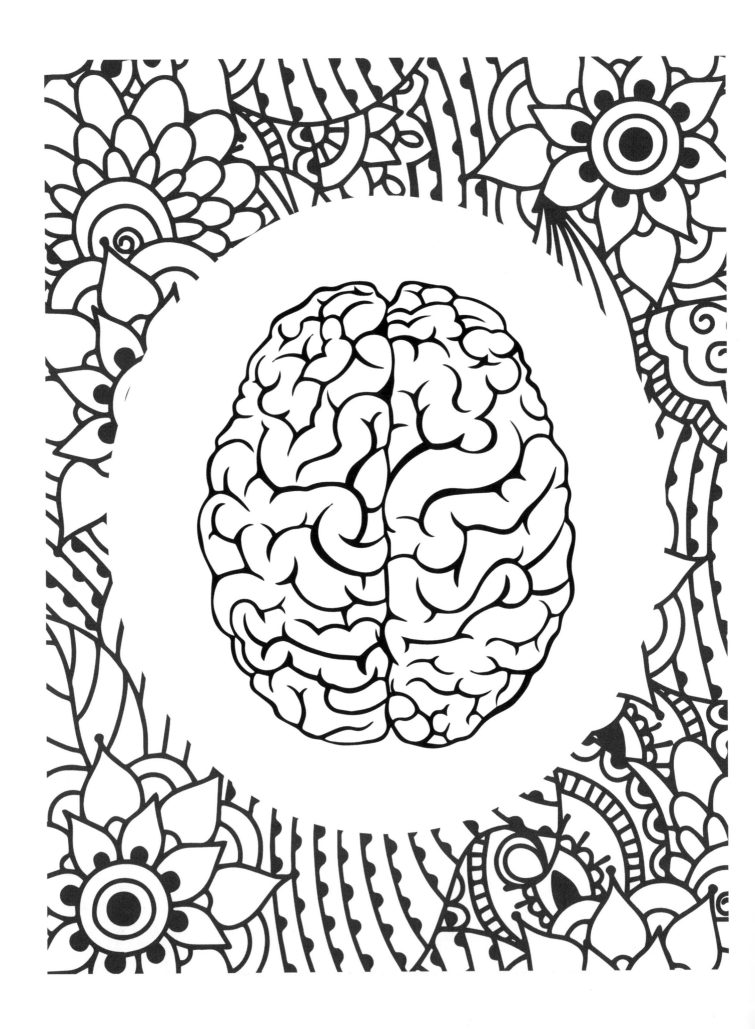

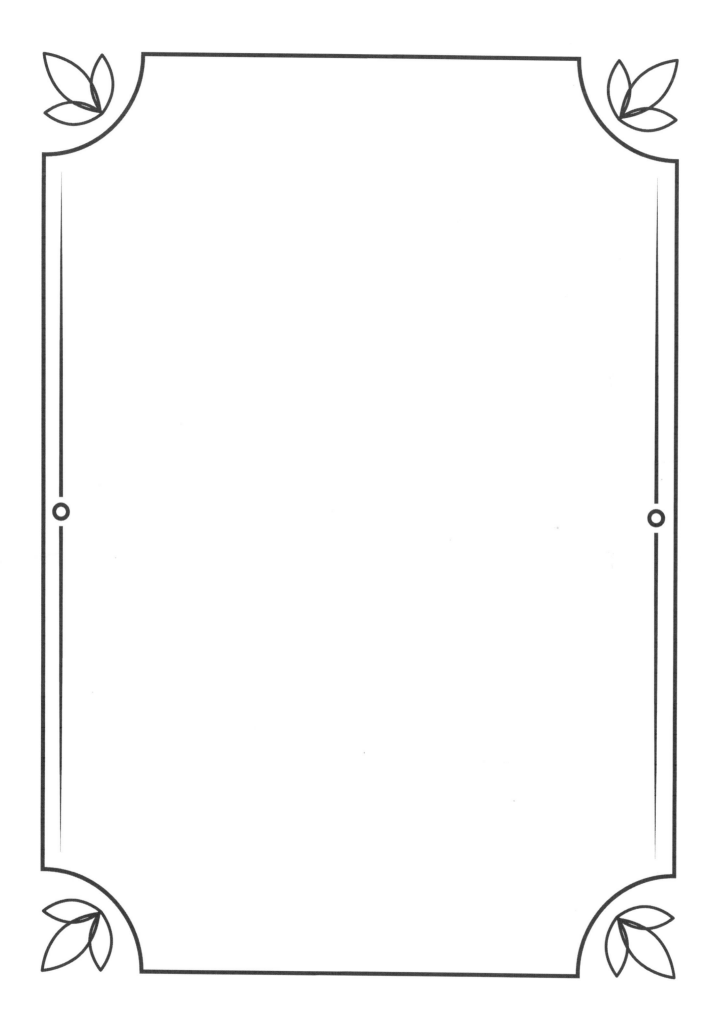

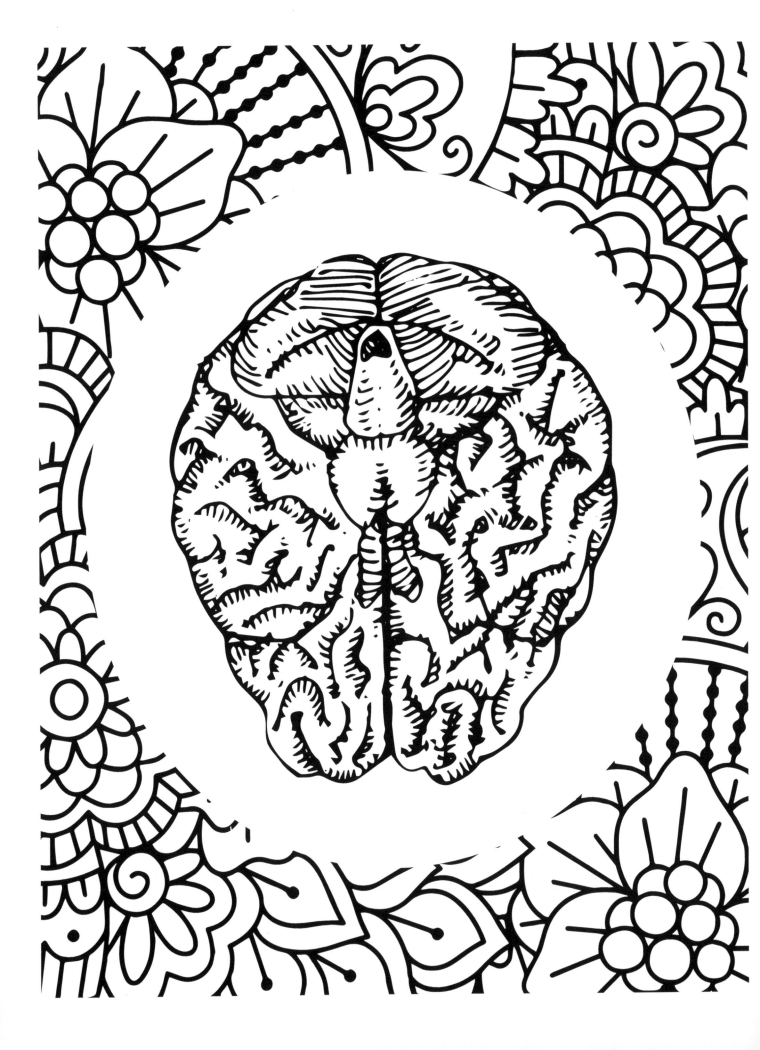

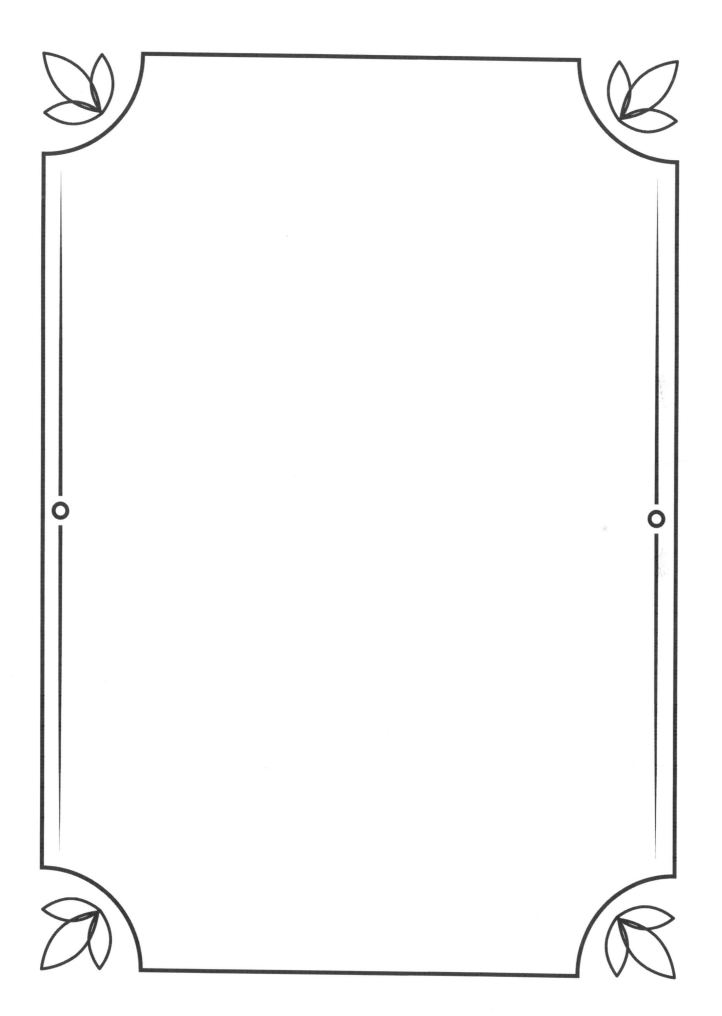

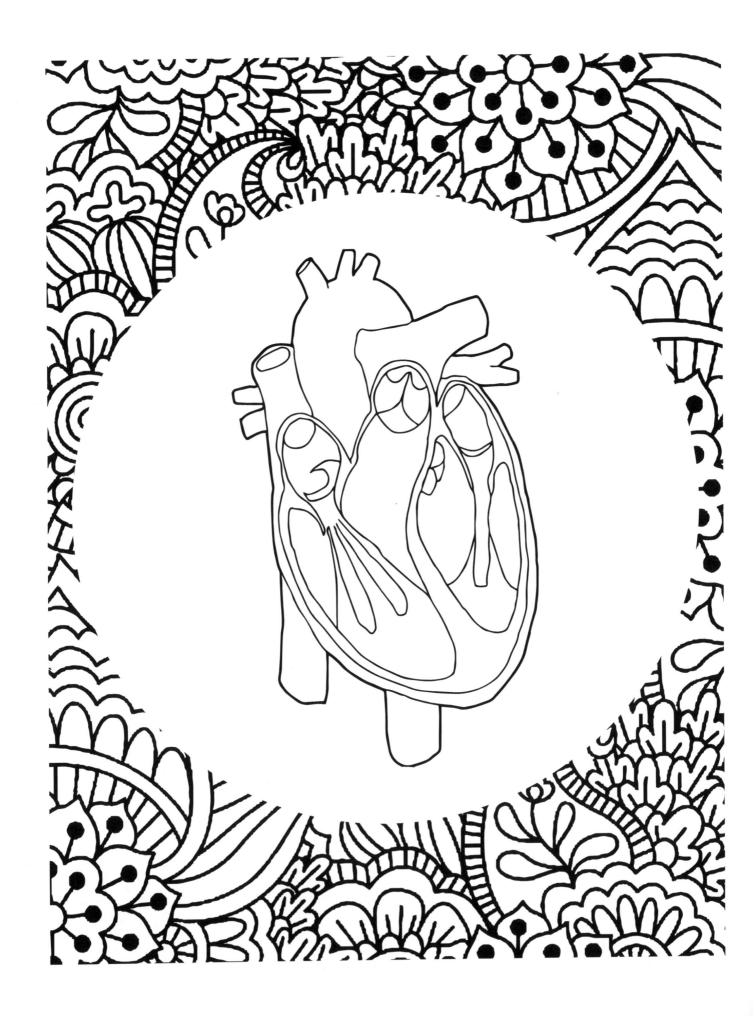

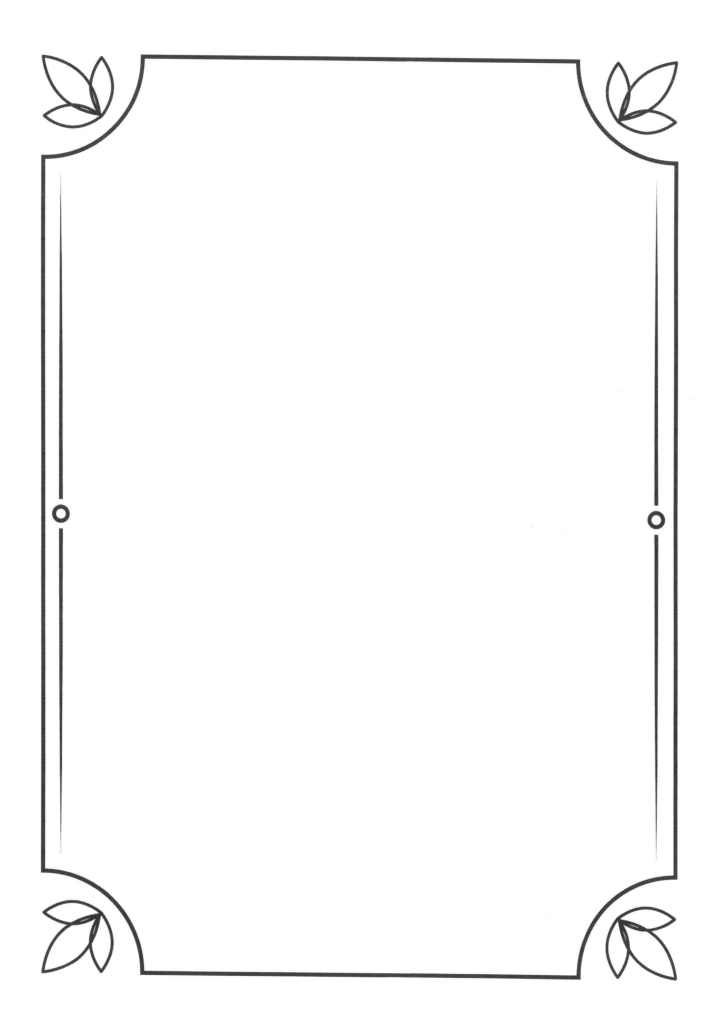

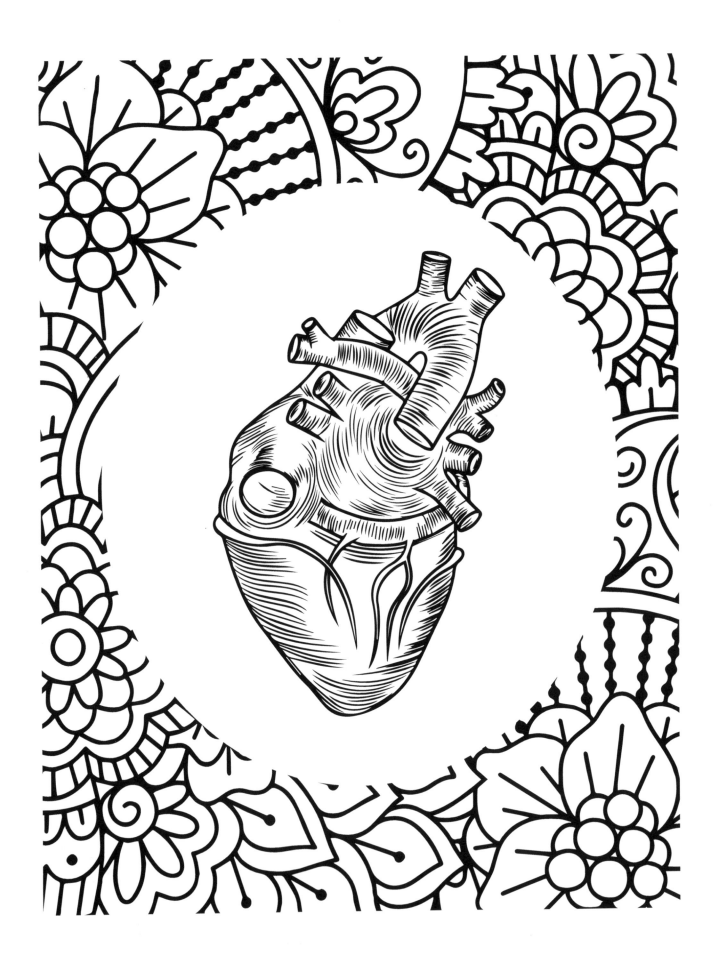

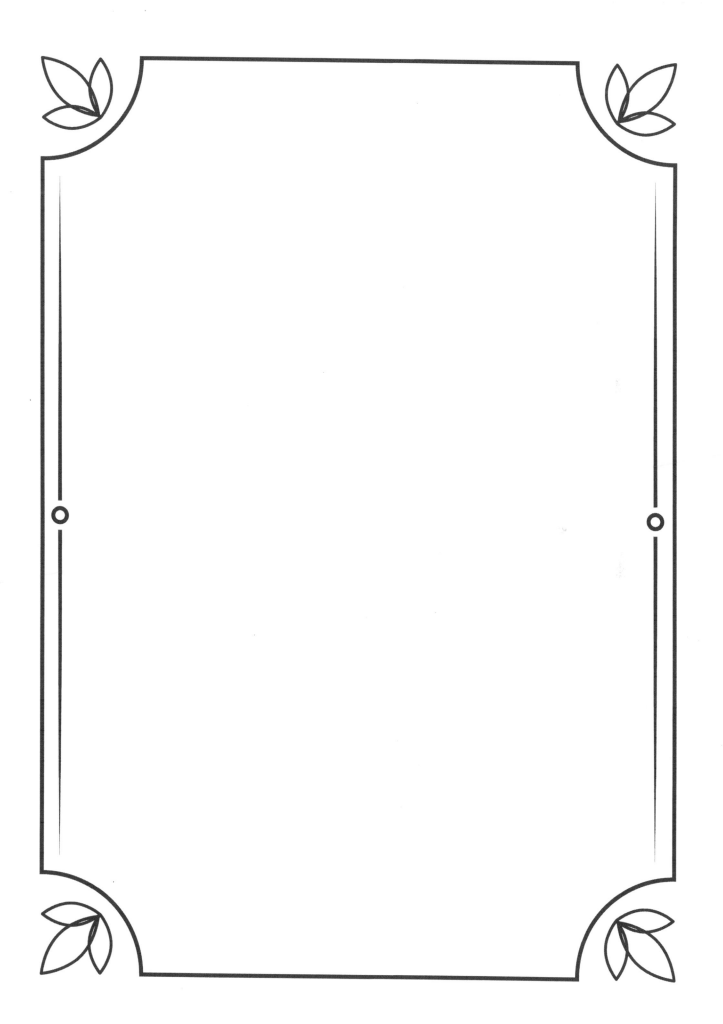

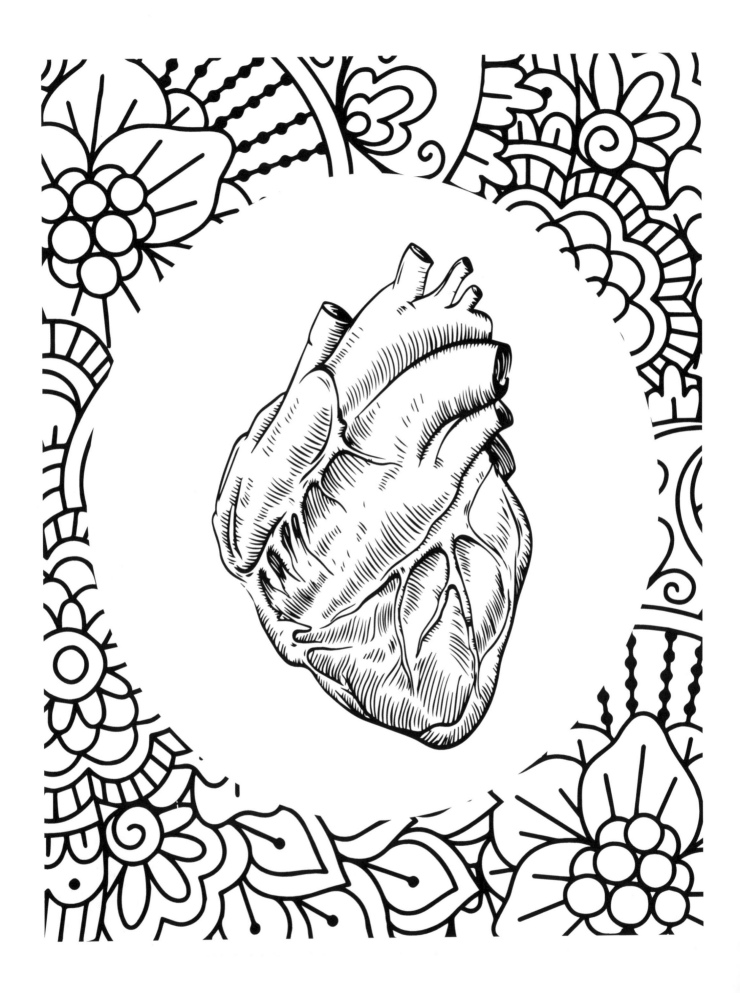

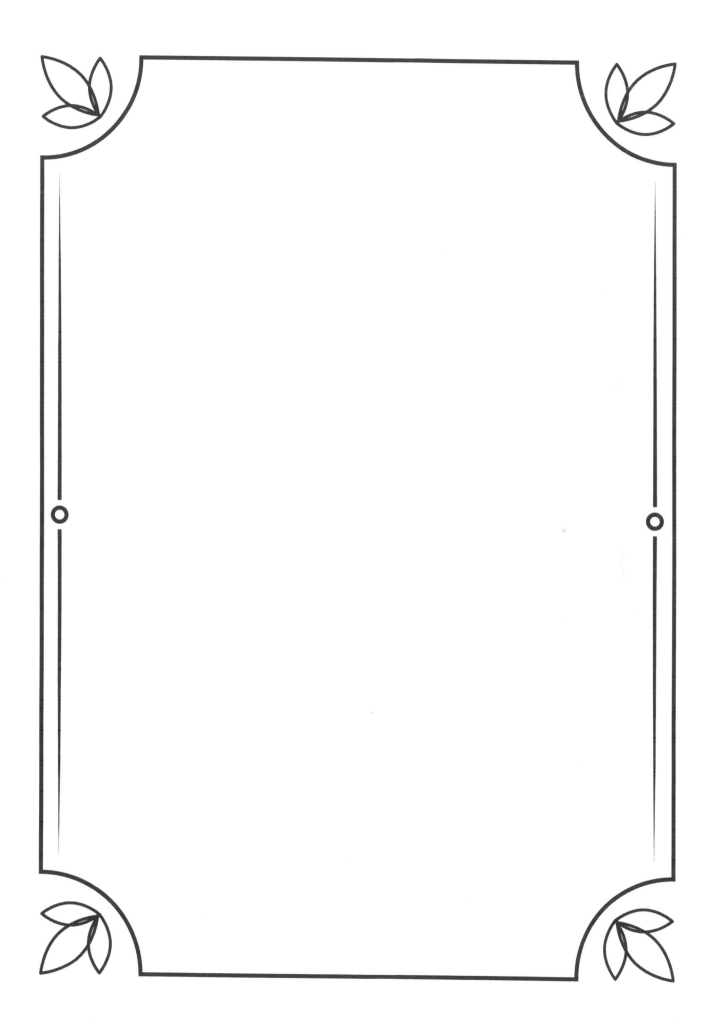

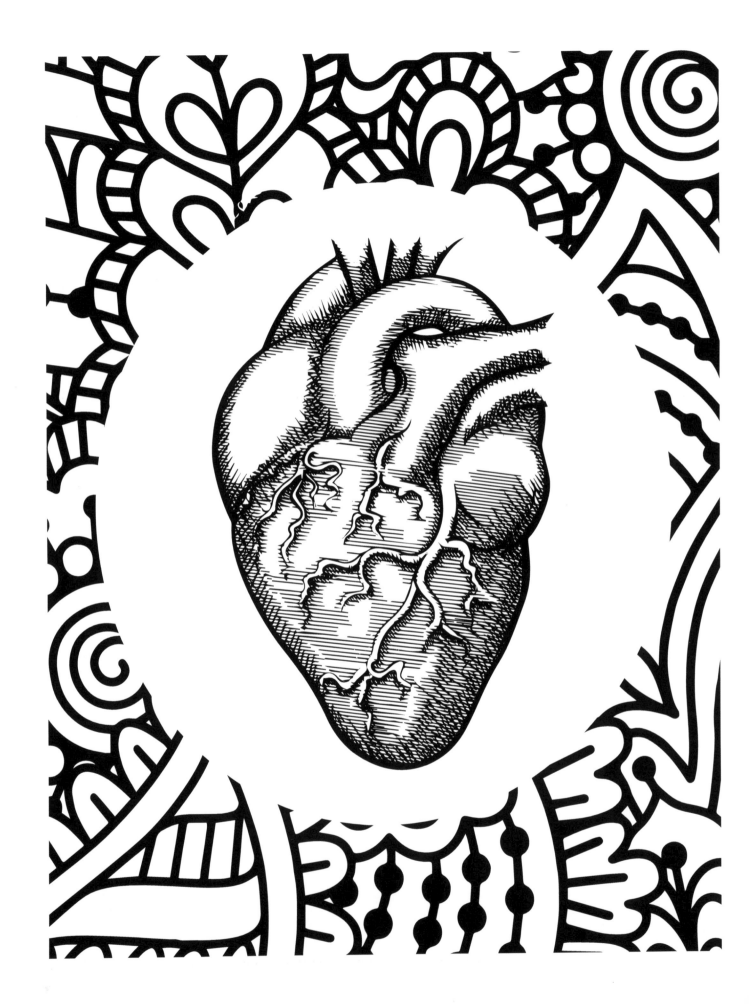

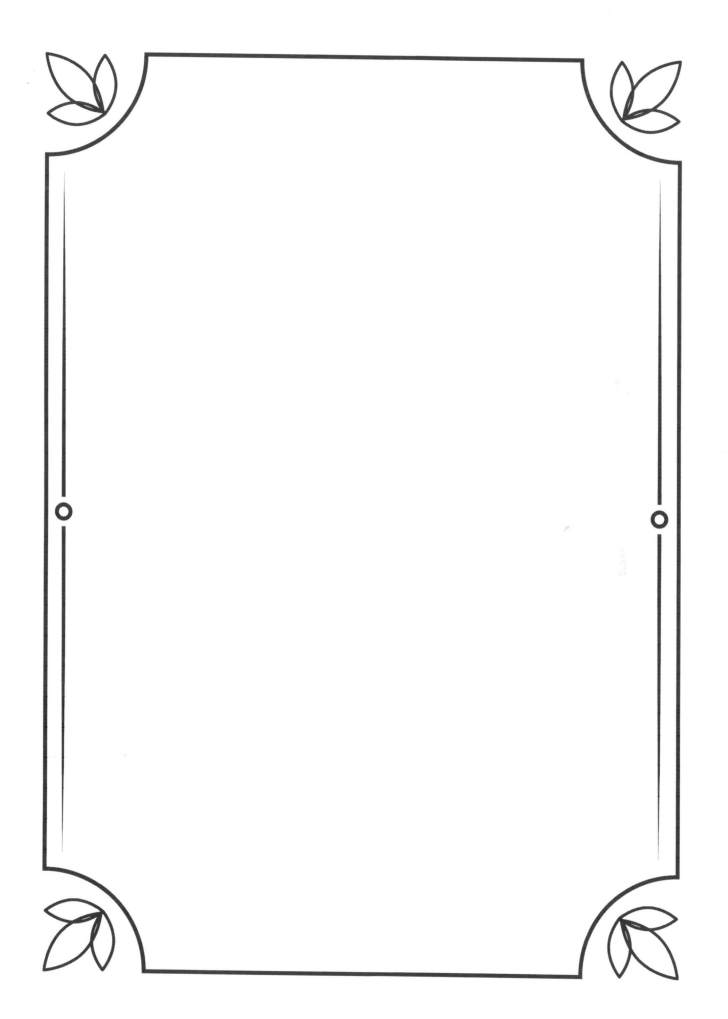

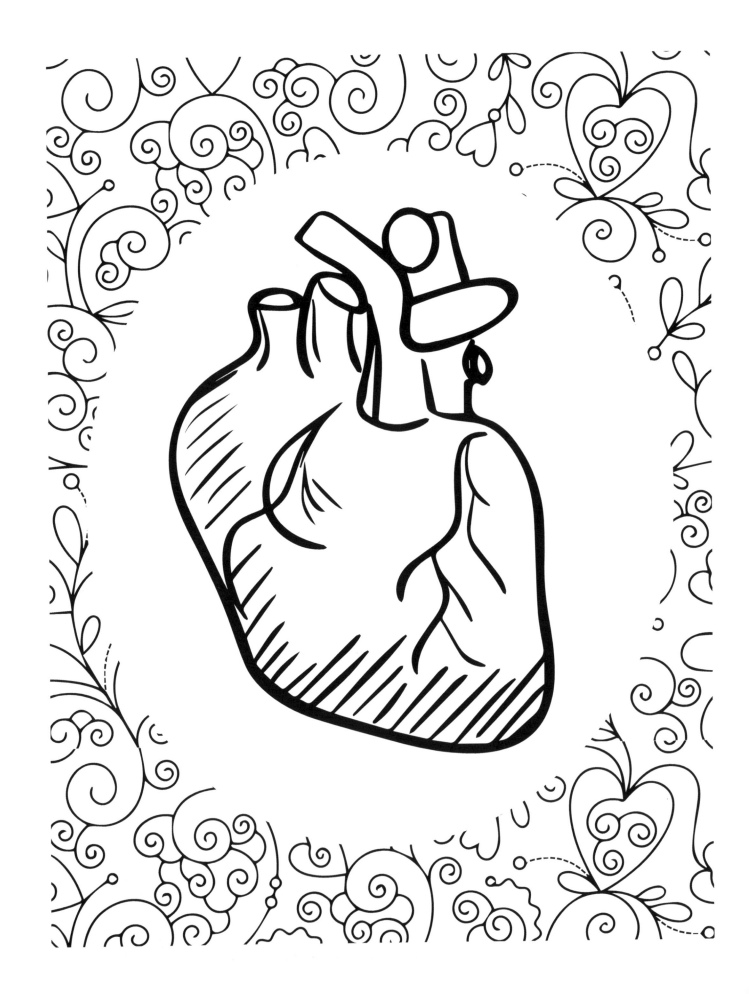

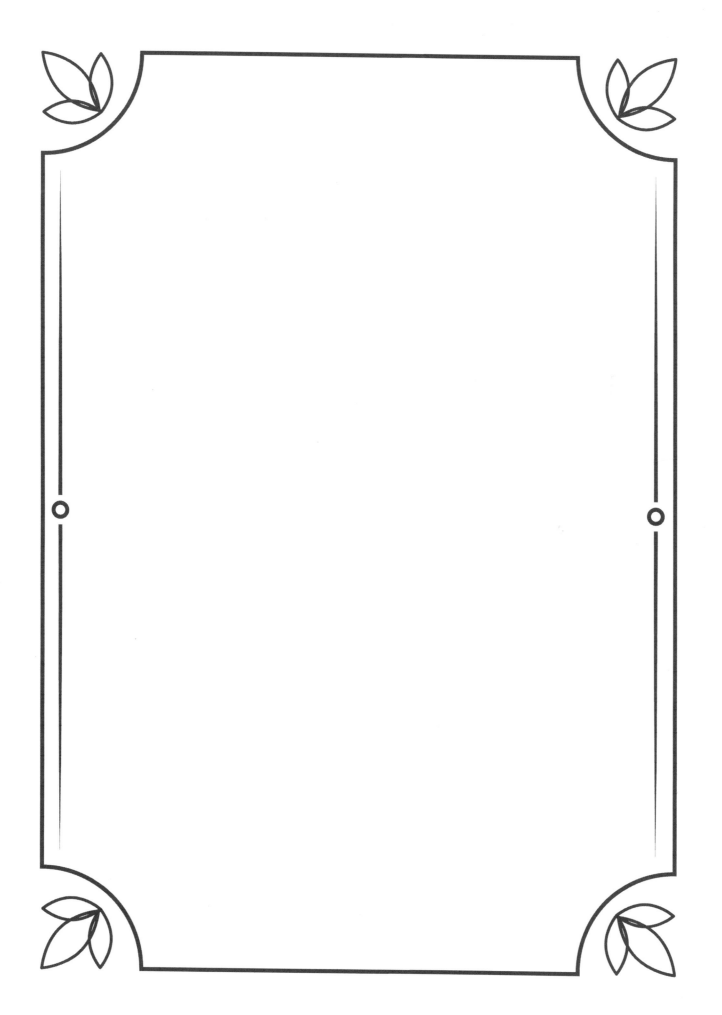

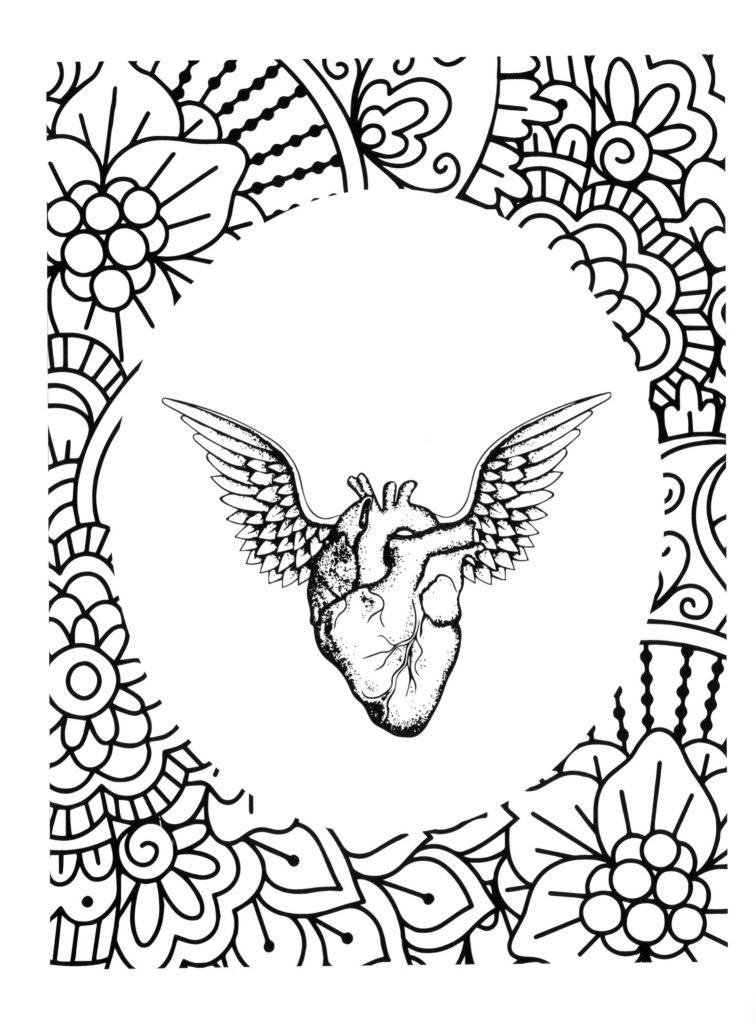

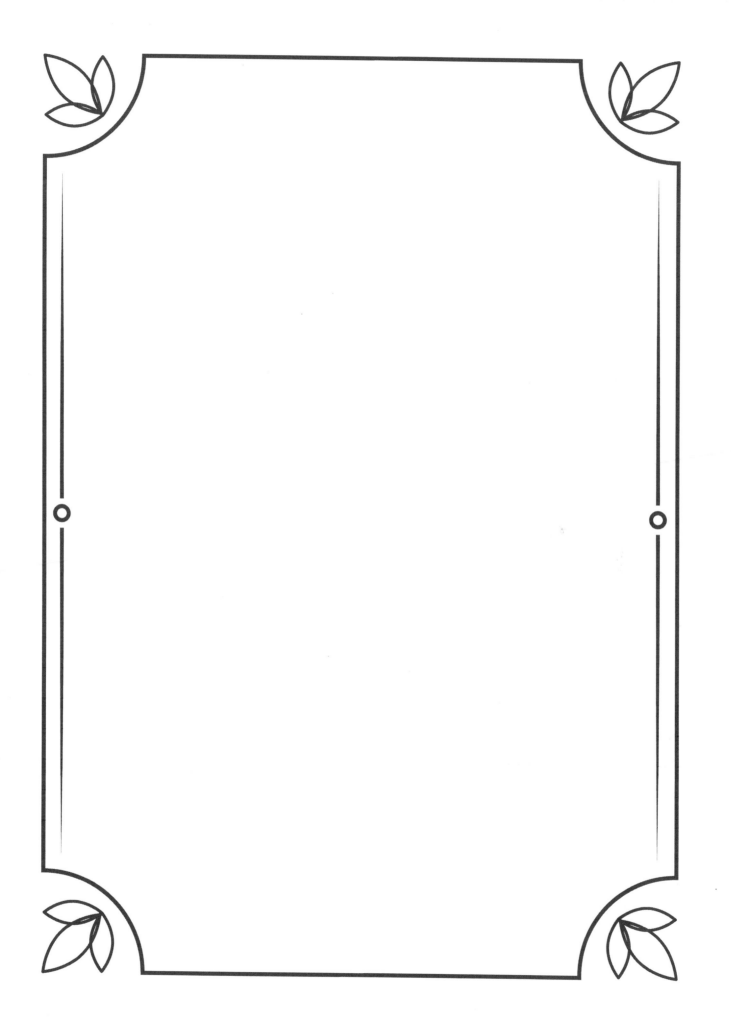

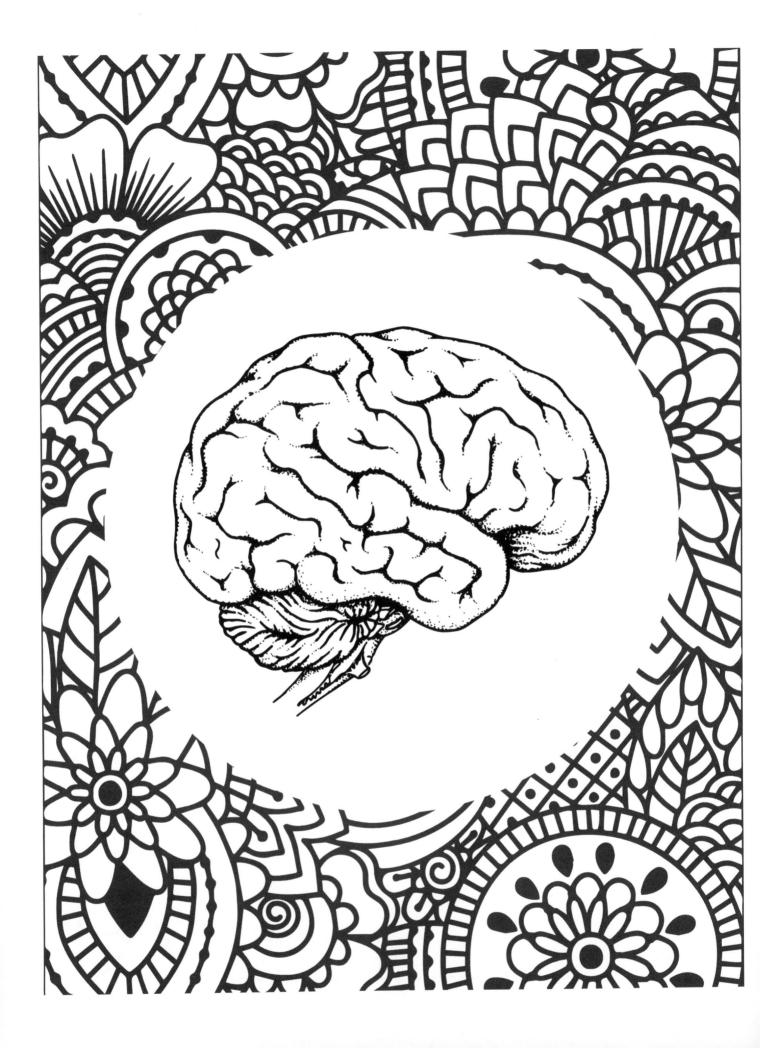

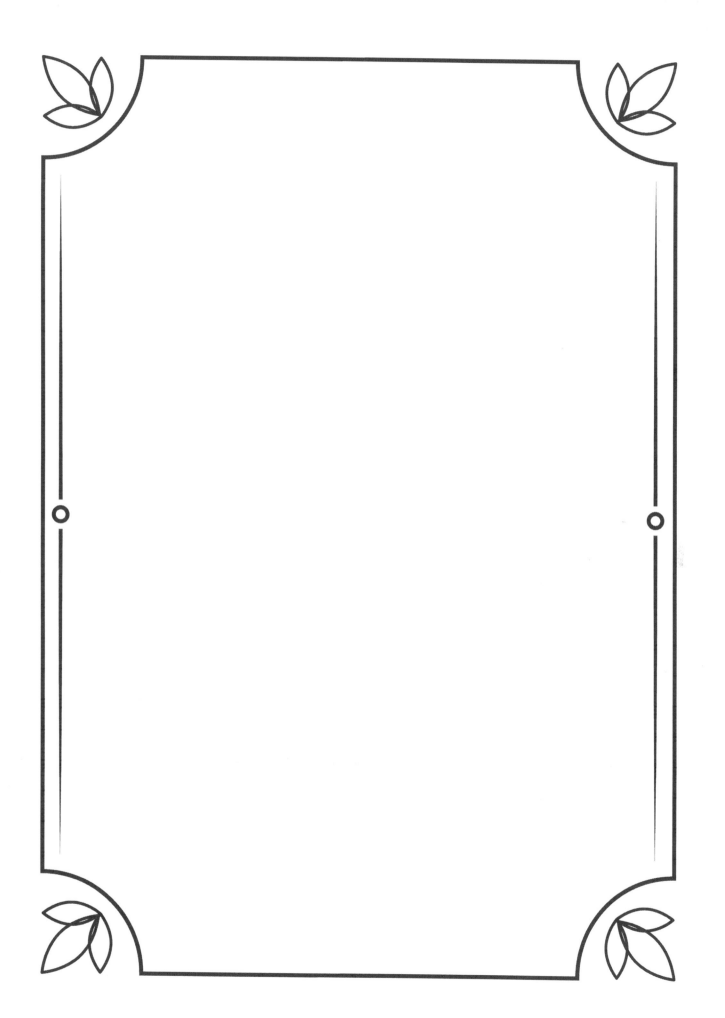

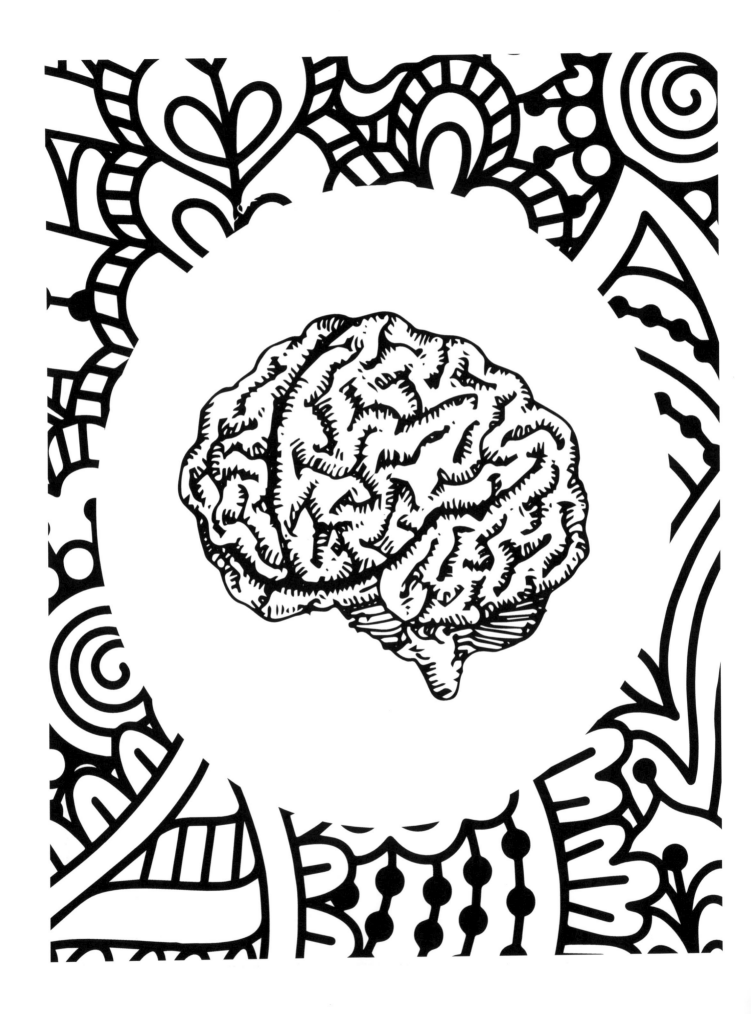

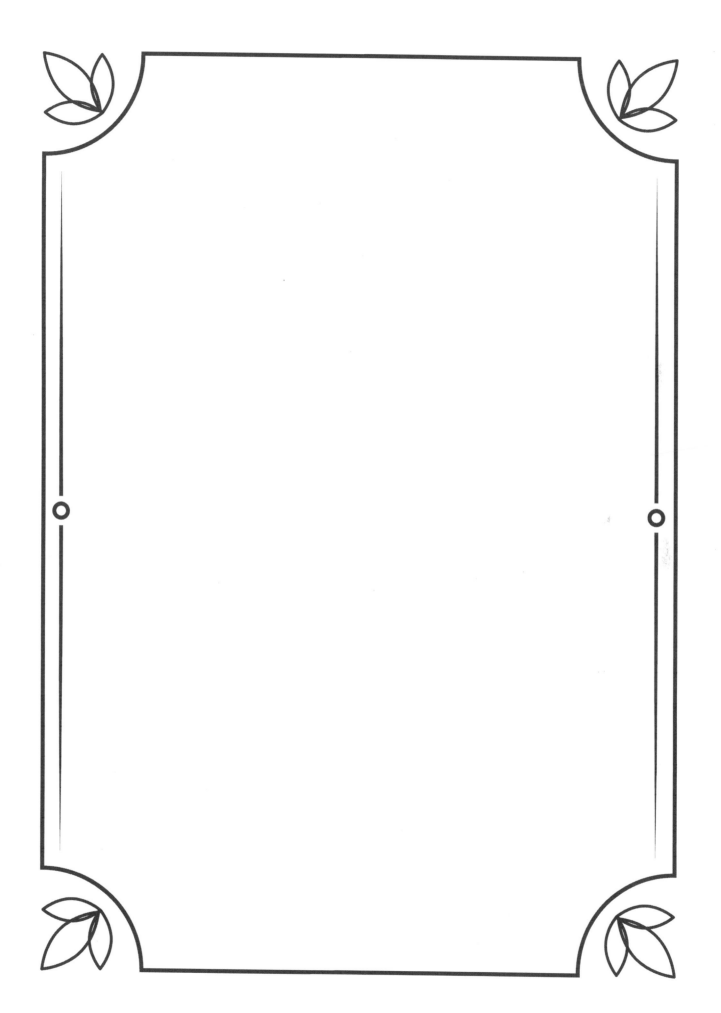

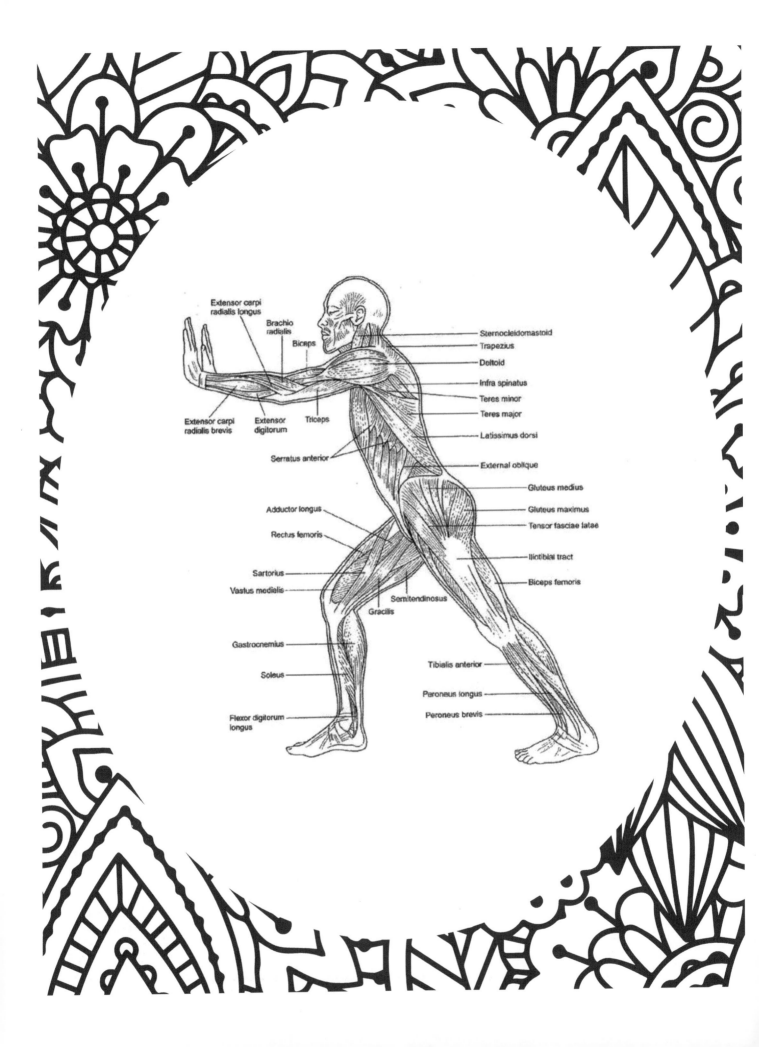

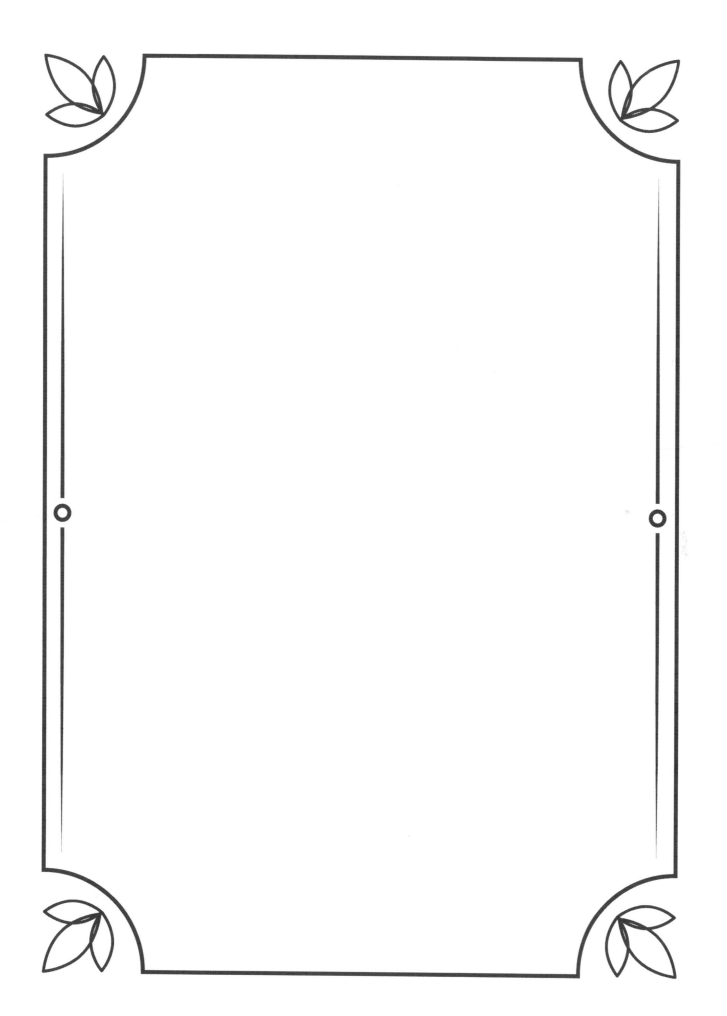

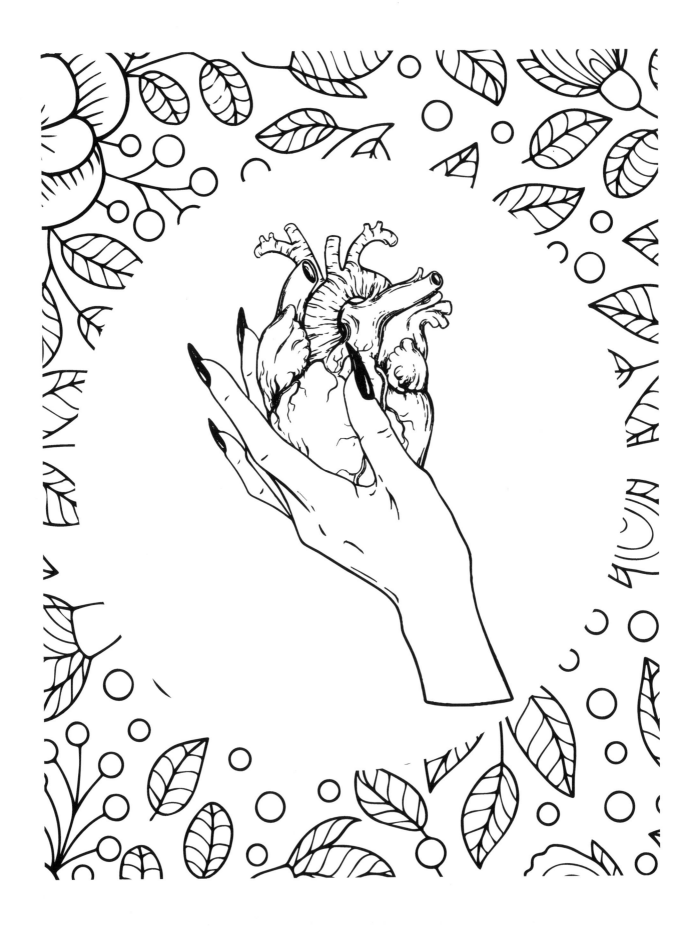

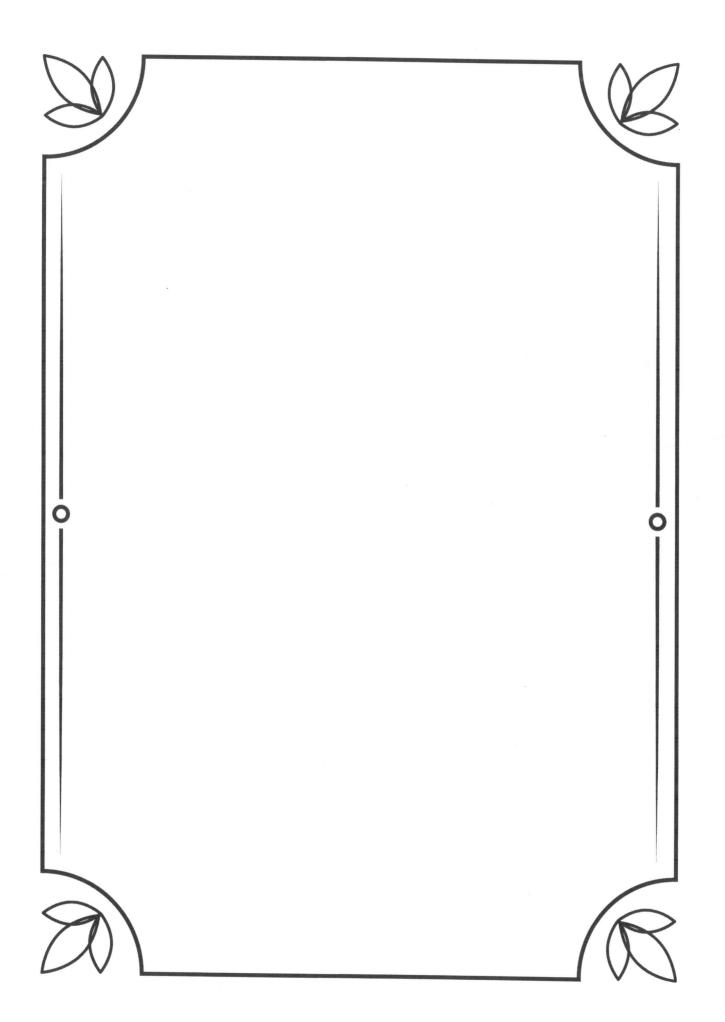

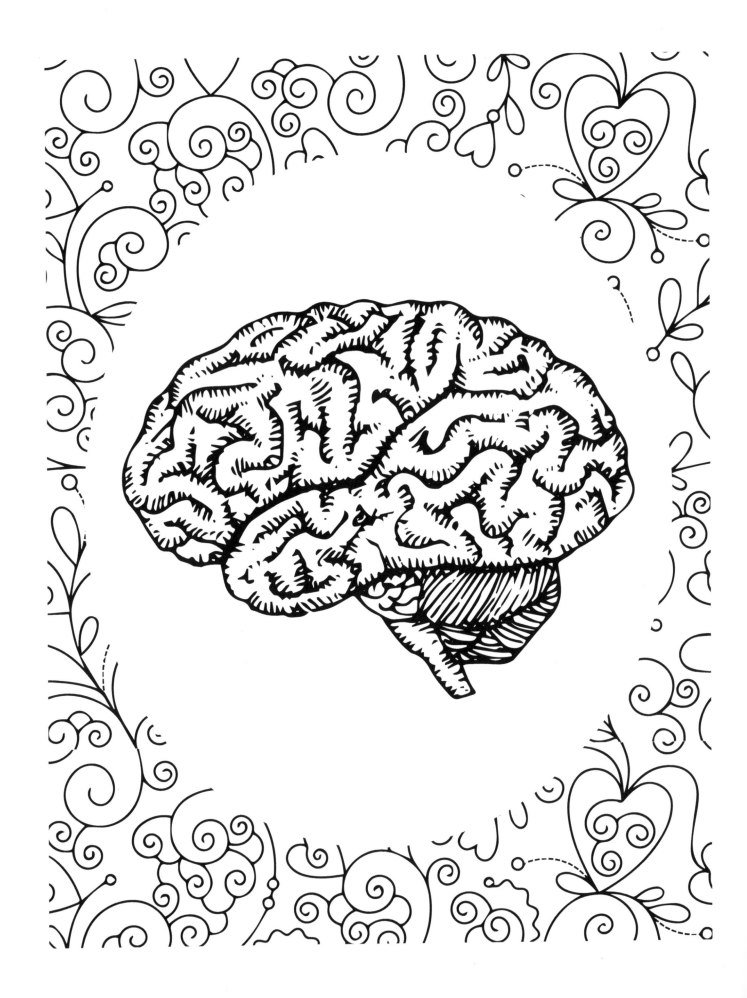

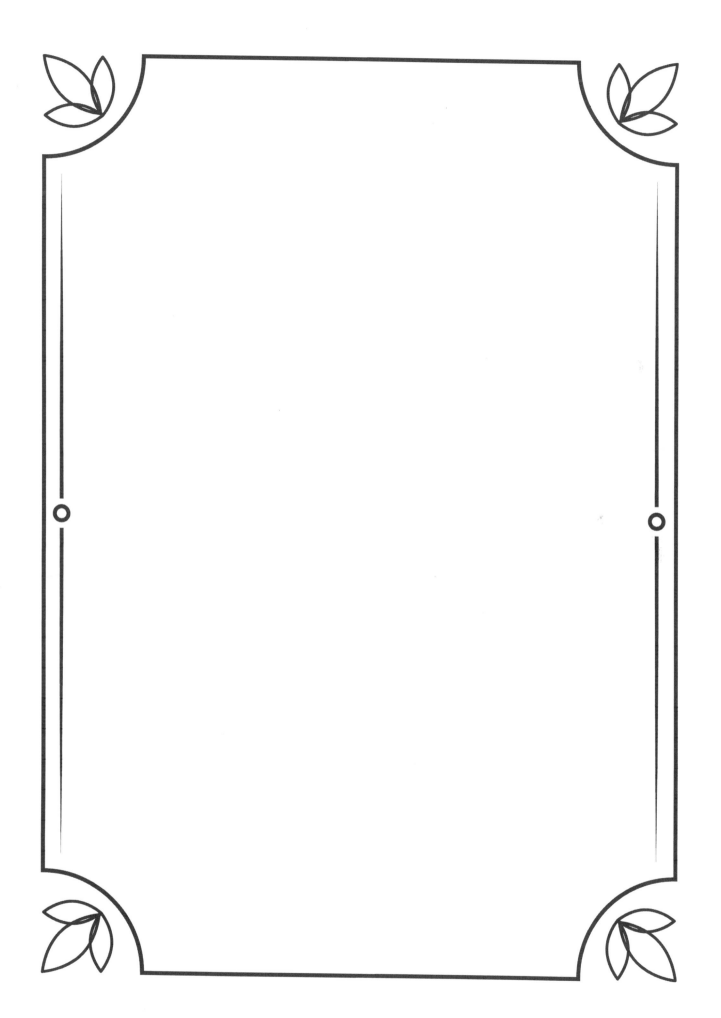

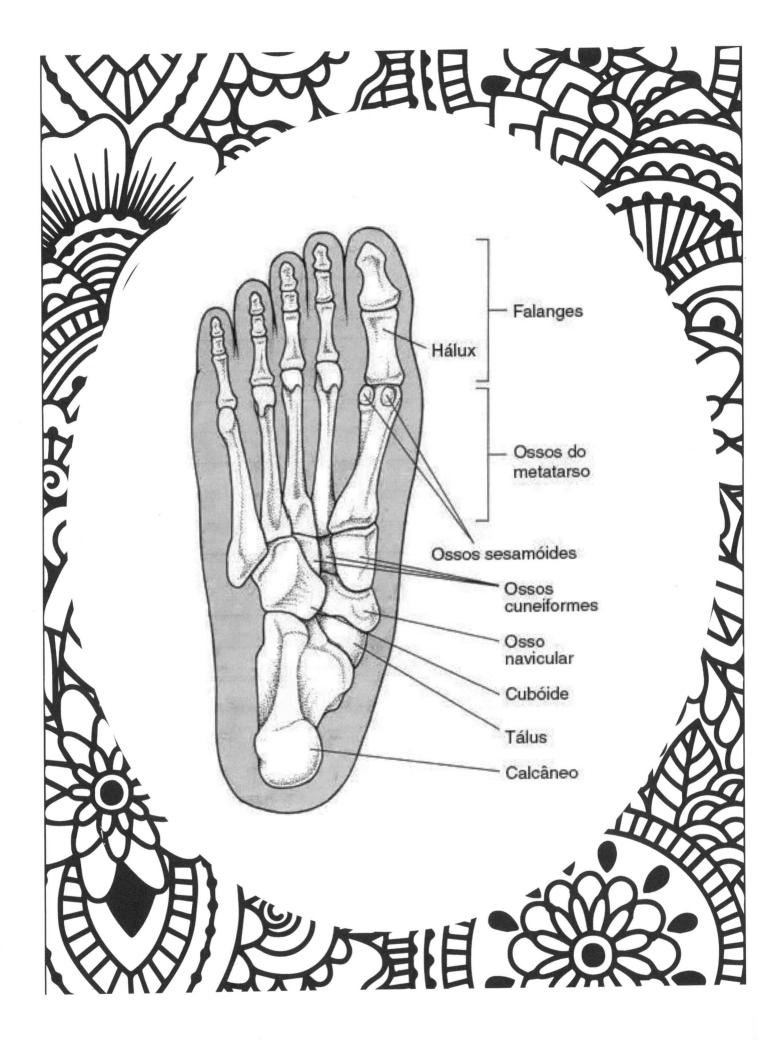

Falanges

Hálux

Ossos do
metatarso

Ossos sesamóides

Ossos
cuneiformes

Osso
navicular

Cubóide

Tálus

Calcâneo

Printed in Germany
by Amazon Distribution
GmbH, Leipzig

21235006R00059